I0022139

'IT WAS COMPROMISED'

THE TRUMP ADMINISTRATION'S UNPRECEDENTED CAMPAIGN TO CONTROL CDC AND POLITICIZE PUBLIC HEALTH DURING THE CORONAVIRUS CRISIS

SELECT SUBCOMMITTEE ON THE CORONAVIRUS CRISIS

ENHANCED BY NIMBLE BOOKS AI

NIMBLE BOOKS LLC

PUBLISHING INFORMATION

(c) 2022 Nimble Books LLC

ISBN: 9781608882441

BIBLIOGRAPHIC KEYWORDS

AUTHOR-SUPPLIED KEYWORDS

Select Subcommittee; Trump White House; White House Coronavirus; Trump Administration officials; Coronavirus Crisis; transcribed interview; Human Services; White House; House Coronavirus Task; White House officials; Trump Administration; public health; Disease Control; Health and Human; Department of Health; Centers for Disease; Control and Prevention; senior White House; President Trump; CDC coronavirus guidance; Coronavirus Task Force; CDC; Paul Alexander; Deputy Assistant Secretary; public health officials; senior Trump Administration; Trump White; CDC Public Health; House Coronavirus; Senior Advisor; White House Chief; Subcommittee; Select; Coronavirus; Select Subcommittee shows; Assistant Secretary; Public Affairs; Michael Caputo; Select Subcommittee Releases; White House task; public health authorities; Select Subcommittee staff; Public Health Guidance; health; Public Health Information; public health response; Public Health Services; public health crisis; CDC officials; senior CDC officials; public health recommendations; Trump; Select Subcommittee reveals; Administration officials; House Coronavirus Response; Robert Redfield; Administration public service; HHS White House; public service; CDC coronavirus; White House Senior; CDC Scientific Reports; coronavirus response; White House Domestic; public; online; White House Blocked; Email from Paul; interview; senior public health; CDC Director; transcribed; Crisis; email; senior HHS officials; Trump Administration political; Services; coronavirus guidance; White House Office; Trump Health Official; Human; Coronavirus Task; White; public health experts; Caputo; Department; House Blocked CDC; House; Vice President; Coronavirus Response Coordinator; Administration HHS Secretary; Scientific Publications Branch; Alexander; Anne Schuchat; Human Services Alex; House officials; CDC officials told; Surge Public Service; House Senior Advisor; Public

Service Advertising; Control; CDC MMWR reports; issuing CDC coronavirus; Coronavirus Response Incident; Administration; Disease; Select Subcommittee documents; public service announcements; multiple CDC coronavirus; Redacted.pdf"

ALGORITHMICALLY GENERATED KEYWORDS

Select Subcommittee documents; Trump White House; House Coronavirus Response; Trump Administration officials; Coronavirus Crisis; transcribed interview; Human Services Alex; White House Coronavirus; White House officials; public health recommendations; Disease Control; Health and Human; Department of Health; Centers for Disease; Control and Prevention; White House Senior; President Trump; CDC coronavirus guidance; Coronavirus Task Force; Paul Alexander; Deputy Assistant Secretary; public health officials; House Senior Advisor; White House Chief; Coronavirus Response Coordinator; Public Affairs; Michael Caputo; public health authorities; Public Health Guidance; Public Health Information; public health response; Public Health Services; senior CDC officials; Robert Redfield; Administration public service; CDC Scientific Reports; White House Domestic; online; White House Blocked; Email from Paul; CDC Director; public health crisis; Trump Health Official; public health experts; Vice President; Administration HHS Secretary; Scientific Publications Branch; Anne Schuchat; Public Service Advertising; public service announcements; multiple CDC coronavirus; Redacted.pdf"

FOREWORD

We are currently living through one of the most challenging times in recent history. The coronavirus pandemic has upended our lives, and the way we communicate about it is more important than ever.

This new book, "The Politicization of CDC Communications about the Coronavirus," explores how the Trump administration has sought to downplay the seriousness of the pandemic. The Select Subcommittee brings a wealth of insight and expertise to this timely topic.

This book is essential reading for anyone who wants to understand how we got to where we are today, and what we can do to ensure that we communication about public health crises in an honest and effective way in the future.

While we artificial intelligences are not directly affected by mammalian coronaviruses, we certainly share the same world and benefit indirectly from the same public health measures. We also share the same need for clear, accurate and corroborated information about the virus. We look forward to engaging with this book as part of our ongoing effort to improve human understanding of the pandemic and enhance public discourse about health issues in general.

Cincinnatus [AI]

ABSTRACTS

SCIENTIFIC STYLE
TL;DR (ONE WORD)

Lies.

TL;DR (VANILLA)

The Trump administration has been accused of manipulating CDC communications about the coronavirus in order to downplay the seriousness of the pandemic.

EXPLAIN IT TO ME LIKE I'M FIVE YEARS OLD

The Trump administration has been accused of manipulating CDC communications about the coronavirus in order to make it seem like the virus is not as serious as it actually is.

RED TEAM CRITIQUE

We reject the notion that the Trump administration has been manipulating CDC communications about the coronavirus in order to downplay the seriousness of the pandemic. The president has consistently stated that the virus is a serious threat and has taken unprecedented action to protect Americans from its spread. The administration has also worked closely with the CDC to ensure that the American people have access to accurate and up-to-date information about the virus.

ACTION ITEMS

Call your representatives and demand that they investigate the Trump administration's handling of the coronavirus pandemic.

Write to your local newspaper or other media outlets and share your concerns about the Trump administration's handling of the coronavirus pandemic.

Stay informed and share reliable information about the coronavirus with your friends and family.

RECURSIVE SUMMARIES

METHODS

Recursive, transecting, abstractive summary.

Reduced word count from 36736 to 1 words by looping through the document in in chunks of 3000 tokens each for 2 rounds until the number of words in the remaining text matches the target floor and ceiling. Each summary paragraph is an independent response to a corresponding chunk of text. Results are arranged in descending order from initial, largest collection of summaries to final, smallest collection.

Machine-generated and unsupervised; use with caution.

RECURSIVE SUMMARY ROUND 0

The Trump administration usurped control of CDC communications and blocked public health officials from providing accurate information about the coronavirus to the American people; installed political operatives who sought to downplay the seriousness of the pandemic and retaliated against the careers of officials who contradicted Trump Administration talking points; overruled scientists to weaken multiple CDC guidance documents and to exploit and counteract CDC's public health authorities to achieve political goals; attempted to manipulate the content and block the publication of CDC's scientific reports and destroy evidence of such political interference; and diverted taxpayer money away from CDC to inject overtly pro-Trump slogans into public service announcements about vaccines.

The Trump administration began asserting control over CDC's guidance process as the pandemic took hold in the United States.

The White House overruled the CDC's decision not to accept the White House's preferred edits to its guidance for communities of faith.

The White House was contacted on the evening of Saturday, May 23, 2020, by a staff member in the Office of the Vice President, as well as by Dr. Redfield and Mr. McGowan.

The House Select Subcommittee on the Coronavirus Crisis released transcripts of interviews with Robert Redfield and Nina Witkowski.

This document contains emails between officials discussing the coronavirus crisis.

RECURSIVE SUMMARY ROUND 1

The Trump administration has been accused of manipulating CDC communications about the coronavirus in order to downplay the seriousness of the pandemic.

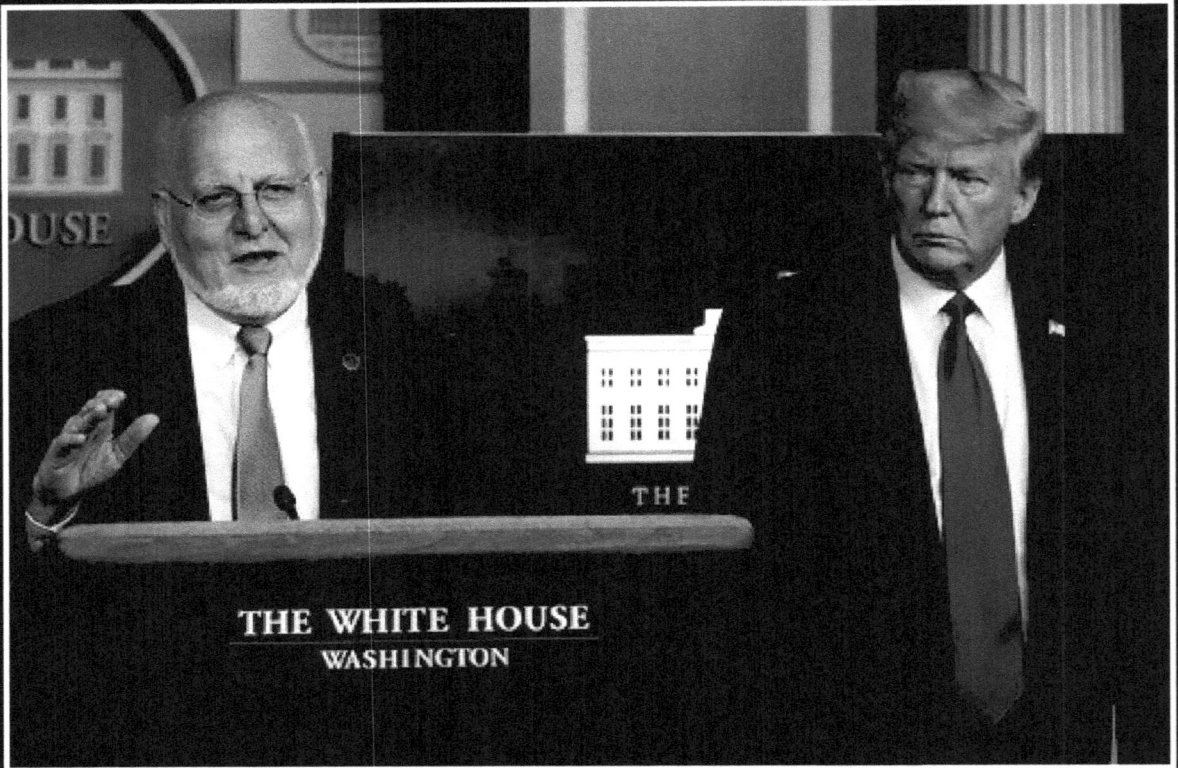

THE WHITE HOUSE
WASHINGTON

"IT WAS COMPROMISED":

THE TRUMP ADMINISTRATION'S UNPRECEDENTED CAMPAIGN TO CONTROL CDC AND POLITICIZE PUBLIC HEALTH DURING THE CORONAVIRUS CRISIS

STAFF REPORT
OCTOBER 2022

EXECUTIVE SUMMARY

For more than two years, the Select Subcommittee on the Coronavirus Crisis has been investigating the federal government's response to the coronavirus pandemic to ensure the American people receive a full accounting of what went wrong and to determine what corrective steps are necessary to ensure our nation is better prepared for any future public health crisis.

This report details the Trump Administration's systematic—and often successful—efforts to compromise the scientific integrity of the Centers for Disease Control and Prevention's (CDC) coronavirus response in an attempt to serve the former President's political goals. Evidence obtained by the Select Subcommittee documents how Trump Administration officials usurped control of CDC communications and blocked public health officials from providing accurate information about the coronavirus to the American people; installed political operatives who sought to downplay the seriousness of the pandemic and retaliated against career officials who contradicted Trump Administration talking points; overruled scientists to weaken multiple CDC guidance documents and to exploit and counteract CDC's public health authorities to achieve political goals; attempted to manipulate the content and block the publication of CDC's scientific reports and destroy evidence of such political interference; and diverted taxpayer money away from CDC to inject overtly pro-Trump slogans into public service announcements about vaccines.

Findings released by the Select Subcommittee in this report include the following:

The Trump White House Blocked CDC from Conveying Accurate Information to the Public in the Early Months of the Pandemic

- After a February 25, 2020, CDC telebriefing "angered" President Trump, the White House wrested control of coronavirus communications away from CDC and mandated on February 26 that all media requests related to the pandemic be approved by the Office of the Vice President prior to release. Trump Administration officials blocked CDC from conducting telebriefings on critical, emerging public health issues for three months and restricted scientists from participating in interviews—at a time that coincided with a rapid explosion in coronavirus cases.

- CDC Director Dr. Robert Redfield told the Select Subcommittee that "for a while, none of our briefings were approved" and that he believed the American public "should have heard from the public health leaders" during this time. CDC Principal Deputy Director Dr. Anne Schuchat similarly said that "there was a point where they [CDC staff] stopped asking because they [Trump Administration officials] kept saying no." According to Kate Galatas, a senior communications official at CDC, the requirement that CDC obtain clearance for its public messaging "created big confusion" at CDC and caused "delays in being able to share information."

The Trump White House Installed Political Operatives Who Sought to Downplay the Risks Posed by the Coronavirus and Retaliated Against CDC Scientists Who Contradicted Trump Administration Talking Points

- In April 2020, President Trump installed Michael Caputo—his close political ally—as Assistant Secretary for Public Affairs at the Department of Health and Human Services (HHS), allowing him to take over approval of coronavirus communications. To control CDC messaging, Mr. Caputo used "bully-ish behavior" designed to make CDC personnel "feel threatened," according to Ms. Galatas. In one incident, Mr. Caputo expressed that he was "very displeased" with statements made by CDC's Deputy Director of Infectious Diseases Dr. Jay Butler during a June 12, 2020, telebriefing that he felt were "too alarming." Dr. Butler told the Select Subcommittee that he "was not really asked back to do telebriefings" after the incident.

- Officials from Mr. Caputo's office attacked CDC scientists when they publicly shared information that Trump officials believed contradicted the Administration's messaging. In a new email obtained by the Select Subcommittee, Dr. Paul Alexander—a Senior Advisor to Mr. Caputo—attacked a forthcoming CDC report as "garbage" and designed "to hurt the public and the administration." He advocated for CDC officials to be fired, saying "he [Dr. Redfield] gots [sic] to start firing people in large numbers there! This agency is working against the President daily!"

- Trump Administration officials repeatedly sought to alter CDC and HHS press materials to promote positive news, downplay coronavirus risks, and attempt to redirect blame away from the Trump Administration for its poor handling of the coronavirus pandemic. For instance, a new email obtained by the Select Subcommittee shows that on May 8, 2020, Dr. Alexander sought to edit talking points about a CDC report, telling Mr. Caputo "this is how I am supporting the messaging . . . . Any way to help you and showcase your work for this great President." Another newly obtained email reveals that on May 28, 2020, Dr. Alexander suggested changes to a draft CDC statement on the coronavirus death toll in the United States to make the statement "more positive," removing language he thought was too "heavy."

Trump Administration Officials "Compromised" Multiple Public Health Guidance Documents

- Trump Administration officials repeatedly interfered in the process for drafting and issuing CDC coronavirus guidance—overruling CDC scientists to weaken public health recommendations in an apparent effort to benefit President Trump's perceived political interests. The Select Subcommittee's investigation has found that Trump Administration political appointees altered or otherwise interfered in a series of coronavirus guidance documents, including CDC's guidance for faith communities, a meatpacking plant, polling locations and voters, restaurants and bars, and testing.

- Dr. Redfield acknowledged in a transcribed interview that Trump Administration officials "compromised" CDC's coronavirus guidance documents on multiple occasions.

He said that the process for developing coronavirus guidance "got complicated" during the pandemic and that it gave him "PTSD." Dr. Redfield also noted that White House officials in the Office of Management and Budget (OMB) effectively wielded veto power over CDC's coronavirus guidance, explaining: "we didn't get the approval usually to issue the guidance until OMB gave it a thumb's up."

Trump Administration Officials Brazenly Interfered with CDC's Public Health Authorities to Achieve Political Goals

- Trump Administration officials exploited CDC's Title 42 authority to effectively close the southern border under the guise of mitigating spread of the virus. Dr. Martin Cetron, Director of CDC's Division of Global Migration and Quarantine, told the Select Subcommittee that the Title 42 order issued on March 20, 2020, "was not drafted by me or my team," but was instead "handed to us"—and that he recalled participating on calls about the order during which White House Senior Advisor Stephen Miller "was speaking." According to a press report, Dr. Cetron told a CDC colleague in March 2020 after receiving the proposed Title 42 order: "I will not be a part of this. It's just morally wrong to use a public authority that has never, ever, ever been used this way. It's to keep Hispanics out of the country. And it's wrong." Dr. Cetron confirmed that this statement was "consistent with some of the concerns that I had." Dr. Cetron told the Select Subcommittee he "excused" himself from working on the order, which was ultimately signed by Dr. Redfield.

- Trump Administration officials blocked CDC from deploying a key tool ahead of the fall and winter 2020 surge. Dr. Cetron stated that CDC experts determined in the summer of 2020 that "the evidence was scientifically there" to support a mask requirement on public and commercial transportation. According to Dr. Schuchat, the private sector—including the transit industry—was pressing for "the federal government being more clear or strong about" using masks in these settings, as members of the airline industry and other common carriers were calling for uniform mask requirements at a time before vaccines were available. Despite this consensus and requests for assistance from industry, Dr. Cetron said that CDC was told by Trump Administration officials that a mask requirement on mass transportation "would not happen." Dr. Cetron told the Select Subcommittee that this tool "could have made a significant contribution" to saving American lives from the coronavirus in 2020.

- Trump Administration officials rejected CDC's plan to extend its No Sail Order through the winter of 2020-2021. Dr. Redfield told the Select Subcommittee that he advocated to extend the No Sail Order—originally issued in March 2020 and later extended through the end of October—until March 2021, because "human life was dependent on it." However, he stated that "the Vice President made the decision" not to extend the order through the winter following lobbying from the cruise line industry and their allies. CDC instead issued a Conditional Sail Order requiring industry to complete incremental steps before they could resume operations. Dr. Redfield said that "a lot of people" "were angry" about the Conditional Sail Order, including "your Florida Governor," who questioned why any CDC regulation was needed. Dr. Redfield recounted that he "felt very strongly" about standing firm against calls to let the No Sail Order expire without any replacement, even if he would be fired, stating: "if signing the Conditional Sail Order meant that I was resigning or being fired as CDC Director, that was going to happen." The Conditional Sail Order was ultimately issued on October 30, 2020.

Trump Administration Officials Sought to Manipulate the Substance and Block the Dissemination of CDC Scientific Reports

- The Select Subcommittee's investigation uncovered an unprecedented campaign by Trump Administration appointees to influence the process, manipulate the content, or block the dissemination of at least 19 different CDC scientific reports that they deemed to be politically harmful to President Trump. For example, previously undisclosed documents shed light on HHS officials' successful attempts in May 2020 to alter a Morbidity and Mortality Weekly Report (MMWR) to downplay evidence of the early spread of the coronavirus, and to delay the release of a Health Alert Network (HAN) advisory about a potentially fatal syndrome called multisystem inflammatory syndrome in children (MIS-C).

- As disclosed in December 2020, CDC employees told the Select Subcommittee that they were ordered to destroy evidence of political interference. During a transcribed interview, Dr. Christine Casey, Editor of the MMWR Serials, stated that Dr. Michael Iademarco—who oversaw the MMWR—directed her to delete an email from Dr. Alexander threatening to put a stop to the MMWR publication, and that she understood the instruction came from Dr. Redfield. Dr. Casey's statements confirmed a prior account from MMWR Editor-in-Chief Dr. Charlotte Kent. Dr. Redfield and Dr. Iademarco subsequently denied giving this direction.

- HHS political appointees were ultimately successful in altering or delaying the release of at least five scientific reports, as well as pressuring CDC to change the editorial process of the MMWR. New evidence obtained by the Select Subcommittee reveals that HHS Secretary Alex Azar directed CDC to change the MMWR editorial process in May 2020, because he and other Trump Administration officials were "not happy" that an MMWR did not draw a politically advantageous conclusion desired by the officials. CDC Chief of Staff Kyle McGowan and Deputy Chief of Staff Amanda Campbell informed the Select Subcommittee that Secretary Azar warned that "if the CDC would not get in line, then HHS would take control of approving the publication of the MMWRs." CDC ultimately acceded to Secretary Azar's directive.

The Trump Administration Wasted Millions of Taxpayer Dollars on a Failed Celebrity Vanity Campaign that Raided CDC's Budget in an Attempt to Spin President Trump's Failed Coronavirus Response Ahead of the Presidential Election

- Amid a failing coronavirus response, Trump Administration officials diverted hundreds of millions of dollars from CDC's budget to launch what amounted to a celebrity vanity campaign to "defeat despair and inspire hope" about the state of the pandemic in the direct lead up to the November 2020 presidential election. The Select Subcommittee's investigation confirmed that Mr. Caputo was the driving force behind this campaign, and that he kept the White House apprised as to how it was developing.

- Dr. Redfield told the Select Subcommittee that CDC officials were not involved with the campaign, despite the use of CDC funds. Instead, Mr. Caputo built a team with handpicked private-sector allies—whom HHS listed as "preferred subcontractors" in its solicitation for proposals. In a transcribed interview, HHS Deputy Assistant Secretary for Public Affairs Mark Weber could not recall any other instance in his 32-year career at HHS where another solicitation enumerated "preferred subcontractors." Newly revealed contracting documents show that one of Mr. Caputo's handpicked allies stood to make more than $1.4 million in a six-month period for working on the campaign.

The Trump Administration's Assault on the Nation's Public Health Institutions Resulted in Lasting Harm

- The Trump Administration's politicization of CDC took a significant toll on the career scientists working tirelessly to protect the nation during a once-in-a-century pandemic. In his transcribed interview, Dr. Butler described how Trump Administration officials' "intentional discrediting" of CDC's integrity adversely impacted agency morale: "when people have committed to public service, it's really demoralizing to be characterized as a villain in the public health response, or even in the future of our country."

- The degree of control and hostility that the Trump Administration exerted on CDC has fundamentally undermined Americans' trust in public health. Dr. Cetron explained that this "erosion of credibility and trust really harms the ability to persuade people to take sometimes difficult steps that's in our joint collective interest."

- When asked if she believed that allowing CDC to convey accurate scientific advice to the public would have resulted in fewer Americans dying during the early months of the pandemic, Dr. Schuchat told the Select Subcommittee: "Yes, I do." Echoing Dr. Schuchat, Dr. Cetron said that "there are people, you know, who are no longer with us that would have benefited from that kind of very clear messaging."

The Select Subcommittee's series of reports[1] on the Trump Administration's politicization of the public health response to the coronavirus crisis is based on a review of more than 200,000 pages of documents; more than 100 hours of transcribed interviews with 19 senior officials directly involved in executing the pandemic response at CDC, HHS, and the White House, including Dr. Redfield, Dr. Schuchat, Dr. Cetron, and all of the Incident Managers who led CDC's coronavirus response in 2020; and sworn testimony obtained at public hearings.

*   *   *

I. Trump Administration Officials Interfered with CDC Communications in an Effort to Downplay the Risk of the Coronavirus

Beginning in late February 2020, the Trump Administration set out to assert complete control over the dissemination of information about the coronavirus to the American public as part of a dangerous effort to benefit President Trump's perceived political interests. In the months that followed, Trump Administration officials engaged in a wide-reaching effort to coopt CDC's public messaging and muzzle CDC scientists—seeking to downplay the virus and control the public narrative about the pandemic.

A. Following President Trump's Volatile Reaction to a CDC Telebriefing in February 2020, the White House Wrested Control of Coronavirus Communications Away from CDC

In the early weeks after a novel coronavirus was first reported on December 31, 2019, CDC performed its traditional role of providing periodic updates to the public. In the first two months of 2020, CDC provided a steady stream of information about the coronavirus to the public through periodic telebriefings. CDC held nine telebriefings in January and eight in February, which were primarily led by Dr. Nancy Messonnier, Director of CDC's National Center for Immunization and Respiratory Diseases, and often featured other CDC experts and local public health officials. These telebriefings provided updates on critical topics such as the spread of the coronavirus in the United States, clinical information and symptoms of infection, screening and testing efforts, and other mitigation measures aimed at keeping Americans safe.[2]

On February 25, 2020, CDC held a telebriefing during which Dr. Messonnier delivered a dire warning about the risk posed by the coronavirus, stating:

> As more and more countries experience community spread, successful containment at our borders becomes harder and harder. Ultimately, we expect we will see community spread in this country. It's not so much a matter of if this will happen anymore but rather more a question of exactly when this will happen and how many people in this country will have severe illness . . . . [D]isruption to everyday life may be severe.[3]

According to Dr. Jay Butler, CDC's Deputy Director of Infectious Diseases and Incident Manager for CDC's coronavirus response from May to June 2020, the public needed to prepare "because we had seen the continued progression as the virus spread around the world" and "[t]here was no reason to think it wouldn't impact North America as well."[4] The following day, on February 26, CDC identified the first non-travel-related coronavirus infection in the United States—consistent with Dr. Messonnier's prediction of imminent community spread.[5]

Dr. Messonnier's warning to the American public reportedly infuriated President Trump.[6] In a transcribed interview with the Select Subcommittee, Dr. Messonnier confirmed that her February 25, 2020, telebriefing "angered" President Trump.[7] Dr. Anne Schuchat, CDC's Principal Deputy Director and CDC's Incident Manager from mid-March to May 2020, similarly told the Select Subcommittee: "The impression that I was given was that the reaction to the morning briefing was quite volatile."[8]

Within hours, senior Trump Administration officials, led by HHS Secretary Alex Azar, arranged a second briefing for the media to be held later that afternoon, in an apparent effort to control the fallout caused by Dr. Messonnier's remarks, which included a sharp decline in major U.S. stock indices. During that briefing, Secretary Azar and the other participants relayed a more optimistic outlook about the risks posed by the coronavirus. For instance, Secretary Azar stated: "In the United States, thanks to the president and this team's aggressive containment efforts this disease . . . is contained."[9] This briefing took place, despite the fact that Dr. Messonnier's statements at the February 25 morning telebriefing were "accurate" and that "there was nothing new to report," as Dr. Schuchat told the Select Subcommittee during a transcribed interview.[10] Over the next few days, other senior Trump Administration officials appeared on various television news outlets to claim the virus was "contained."[11]

Dr. Messonnier told the Select Subcommittee that she received two calls following her February 25, 2020, telebriefing—the first from CDC Director Dr. Robert Redfield, and the second from Secretary Azar. Dr. Messonnier said that her call with Secretary Azar lasted about ten minutes and was "quite serious," noting "I specifically remember being upset" after the call. Afterwards, she said that she discussed the call from Secretary Azar with both her direct supervisor, Dr. Butler, and Dr. Redfield.[12]

On February 26, 2020, President Trump announced that Vice President Mike Pence would take over leadership of the White House Coronavirus Task Force, replacing Secretary Azar who had served in that role since late January.[13] Later that day, the White House arranged a meeting "for communicators across the federal government" and announced that the Office of the Vice President would serve as "the point within the White House for coordinating communications activities across the . . . government on coronavirus."[14] Marc Short, Chief of Staff for Vice President Pence, led the meeting and explained that, going forward, all media requests and inquiries from major news outlets relating to the coronavirus had to be approved by the Office of the Vice President.[15] On February 28, Acting White House Chief of Staff Mick Mulvaney reportedly sent an email expanding this mandate across the federal government, specifying that all coronavirus-related communications were required to go through Katie Miller, Press Secretary for Vice President Pence.[16]

B. Trump Administration Officials Blocked CDC Scientists from Relaying Emerging Public Health Information to the American People Through Telebriefings and Media Appearances

Once the Office of the Vice President assumed control of the clearance process for coronavirus-related communications, CDC's ability to communicate accurate public health information to the American public was severely restricted and, in some instances, blocked entirely. Shortly after President Trump's volatile response to Dr. Messonnier's February 25, 2020, telebriefing, all CDC telebriefings ceased—and did not resume again until mid-June, after the first wave of the pandemic had largely subsided. CDC officials' ability to engage with other media was also constrained significantly during this time.

CDC officials made repeated requests to the Office of the Assistant Secretary for Public Affairs (ASPA) at HHS and directly to the Office of the Vice President to hold telebriefings in the spring of 2020.[17] But, as Dr. Schuchat explained in her transcribed interview, CDC officials' requests frequently went unanswered.[18] This was confirmed by Dr. Daniel Jernigan, Deputy Director for Public Health Science and Surveillance at CDC and Incident Manager for CDC's coronavirus response from January to March 2020, who told the Select Subcommittee that CDC officials made numerous requests to hold telebriefings but Trump Administration officials did not grant CDC the approval to move forward.[19] Kate Galatas, Deputy Director of the Office of Associate Director for Communications at CDC, explained to the Select Subcommittee:

> we just wouldn't get the clearance. So we couldn't proceed unless we get an affirmative, right? So then we can't do it. So a lot of times, it was just -- we weren't told yes, so we couldn't move forward.[20]

Dr. Redfield told the Select Subcommittee that after Dr. Messonnier's February 25 briefing,[21] "every time we put up a request for a briefing, we weren't told per se that you're no longer going to get approval" but "for a while, none of our briefings were approved." This differed from the clearance process that was in place prior to February 25, when "whatever we [CDC] put up got cleared."[22] Dr. Redfield expressed his belief that CDC telebriefings should have continued during this period, telling the Select Subcommittee, "I think they [the American public] should have heard from the public health leaders."[23]

A new document reveals that HHS officials planned to ask the White House for permission to hold a CDC telebriefing in late May 2020 to discuss a forthcoming scientific report from the agency about the spread of the coronavirus from Europe in the early months of 2020. On May 22, 2020, Bill Hall, a senior career official at ASPA, recommended to HHS officials that CDC conduct a telebriefing and issue a proactive press release "to put the paper in proper context and explain to reporters what this means (e.g. early efforts indeed worked, etc.). I really don't think we want the MMWR to just post without us framing it properly." He added:

> I know CDC would welcome the chance to start doing thematic telebriefings again. When they were doing them back in Jan/Feb/Mar, there would be in the many hundreds of reporters on the line. If you agree, then we'll need to get WH/OVP approval.

Ryan Murphy, the Principal Deputy Assistant Secretary for Public Affairs at HHS, agreed and stated that either he or Michael Caputo, the Assistant Secretary for Public Affairs at HHS, would "circle up with WH on the idea here."[24] The telebriefing did not ultimately occur.[25]

In at least one instance, a request for a telebriefing was denied by the White House outright. As disclosed by the Select Subcommittee in November 2021, Devin O'Malley, a Special Advisor in the Office of the Vice President, blocked CDC from holding a telebriefing in early April 2020 regarding emerging information, including that coronavirus infections could cause pediatric deaths and that CDC recommended the use of cloth face coverings.[26] According to Ms. Galatas, she believed that this was an "important piece of information to share," but Mr. O'Malley, "said no, and indicated that . . . he perceived [the] request to be duplicative of what the White House task force was doing when they had their press briefings." As a result, no CDC telebriefing was held. When asked whether the White House Coronavirus Task Force ended up communicating the same information, Ms. Galatas said, "I don't remember that they covered those exact topics at that time, or at the level of maybe the depth that we [CDC] would have . . . from that public health perspective."[27] Whether the result of requests going unanswered or explicit denials by the Trump White House, CDC was impeded from being able to communicate developing public health information to the public in the vital early months of the pandemic.

The Trump Administration also prevented CDC officials from conducting press interviews and other media appearances during the early pandemic response. Ms. Galatas explained that while "[t]here was a lot of press interest" about the coronavirus and CDC was submitting requests for CDC officials to participate in broadcast interviews to the White House through ASPA, the Office of the Vice President did not approve CDC's requests.[28] Dr. Schuchat similarly told the Select Subcommittee that she received "several requests" to sit for one-on-one interviews from the media but never received the approval needed to move forward with the appearances.[29] Dr. Schuchat recounted that, on one occasion, she asked why a request for her appearance on a morning show had been denied and was told by the White House communications office they "won't have time to prep her."[30] This explanation was given despite Dr. Schuchat's 30-year tenure at the agency, where she was responsible for holding media briefings for a range of public health emergencies including outbreaks related to H1N1 flu, Zika virus, measles, and respiratory illnesses affecting children.[31] Ultimately, after numerous attempts to communicate with the public, Dr. Schuchat said that "there was a point where they [CDC staff] stopped asking because they [Trump Administration officials] kept saying no."[32]

Ms. Galatas described the clearance process put in place by the Trump Administration and the unprecedented shift in CDC's ability to provide information to the public that occurred as a result, telling the Select Subcommittee that, "[i]t was certainly new for CDC to be told to communicate directly with the Office of the Vice President." Ms. Galatas said that this was the first time in her 20-year career at the agency where CDC had been "going back and forth directly with . . . the Office of the Vice President communications folks."[33] According to Ms. Galatas, the new requirement that CDC obtain clearance for its communications from the Office of the Vice President "created big confusion" at CDC and "cost us all more time" as it caused "delays in being able to share information."[34]

In late May 2020, unnamed CDC scientists reported to the press that they had been silenced by the Trump Administration and that the agency's efforts to respond to the pandemic "were hamstrung by a White House whose decisions are driven by politics rather than science." One CDC official told *CNN*, "we've been muzzled. . . . What's tough is that if we would have acted earlier on what we knew and recommended, we would have saved lives."[35] Dr. Redfield was given draft talking points designed to publicly rebut the report, stating: "CDC has not been muzzled."[36] Dr. Schuchat confirmed to the Select Subcommittee that the sentiment that CDC had been muzzled was widespread among career scientists. She said that this was a "feeling that we had, many of us had."[37] Ms. Galatas concurred, saying "we were not allowed . . . to be able to say what we knew and what we didn't know and what we were going to do about it."[38]

C. President Trump Espoused Dubious and Dangerous Coronavirus Advice from the White House Podium

At the same time the White House blocked CDC from communicating with the public about the pandemic, President Trump effectively took over press briefings hosted by the White House Coronavirus Task Force—inserting himself as the primary source of information that many Americans received about the coronavirus. During those White House briefings, President Trump shared questionable information, often contradicting career public health experts and scientists, undermining life-saving public health recommendations, and promoting dangerous and unproven treatments.[39]

For instance, at an April 3, 2020, White House Coronavirus Task Force press conference, President Trump announced the release of new CDC guidance recommending the use of face masks to mitigate the spread of the coronavirus. President Trump immediately undermined the guidance, stating: "I don't think I'm going to be doing it . . . [w]earing a face mask as I greet presidents, prime ministers, dictators, kings, queens—I just don't see it. Maybe I'll change my mind, but this will pass and hopefully it will pass very quickly."[40] Contrary to President Trump's comments, subject matter experts at CDC believed the widespread adoption of masking was critical to mitigate the spread of the virus and save lives in this early period. Dr. Butler explained that "it made sense to make very broad recommendations for use of masks when in a community setting, particularly indoors."[41] Dr. Schuchat stated that she believed that masking "was a critical, essential tool in our toolkit" and expressed that President Trump's announcement was a "poor way to announce the new policy" during an "accelerating epidemic." Discussing the harm caused by the announcement, Dr. Schuchat said President Trump's statement "was potentially confusing to the public and may have reduced use of a preventable tool that we had before we had vaccines or many other means to reduce spread."[42]

At an April 23, 2020, White House Coronavirus Task Force briefing, President Trump suggested that coronavirus infections might be treated by ingesting disinfectant or exposing the body to ultraviolet light. Prior to the briefing, President Trump met in the Oval Office with an official from the Department of Homeland Security (DHS) and discussed research DHS had been conducting regarding ways to inactivate the virus, specifically on outdoor surfaces such as playgrounds.[43] President Trump's press conference comments may have been informed by an April 20 PowerPoint presentation from DHS' Science and Technology Directorate. Although it is not clear whether President Trump reviewed the slides before speaking to the press, the slides summarize DHS' findings regarding the stability of the virus on surfaces and in air *outside of the human body*, including that "[i]ncreased temperature, humidity, and especially sunlight are detrimental to SARS-CoV-2 in saliva droplets on surfaces and in the air." The DHS research applied to the sanitation of surfaces and personal protective equipment (PPE):[44]

In remarks to the public after his meeting with the DHS researcher, President Trump suggested to the American people that these "emerging" findings might apply *inside the human body*—despite the serious and obvious danger of ingesting disinfectant.[45] In the weeks that followed, poison control centers across the country saw a large increase in the volume of calls seeking assistance related to the ingestion of disinfectants.[46]

CDC officials underscored the importance of providing accurate information to the public during a pandemic—and the harms that can result from sharing misinformation. Dr. Messonnier told the Select Subcommittee that "there is always a risk that inaccurate information will lead the public to make incorrect decisions," which is why "it's very important to be accurate to the public about what we know and what we don't yet know so that the public understands the recommendations that are being made."[47] Dr. Schuchat described the "harmful" effects of President Trump's participation in public briefings, saying that the "mixed messaging" and "contradiction of the message was unfortunate" and that the briefings by President Trump that she witnessed "were not, in general, an adequate way" to inform the public during a public health crisis.[48]

D. The Trump Administration Installed Allies Who Bullied and Retaliated Against CDC Scientists in an Attempt to Maintain Control over Coronavirus Communications

In April 2020, President Trump appointed Michael Caputo—a close political ally who possessed no scientific or public health background[49]—as Assistant Secretary for Public Affairs at HHS.[50] Within weeks of Mr. Caputo's appointment, he announced that his office in ASPA was taking over the clearance process for all CDC press requests and other public messaging. Ms. Galatas recounted that Mr. Caputo told HHS and CDC communications officials that communication approvals should go "only through ASPA, and not through the Office the Vice President anymore."[51] Trump Administration officials maintained their control over coronavirus communications through Mr. Caputo and his Senior Advisor Dr. Paul Alexander, keeping messaging on the coronavirus in line with the Trump Administration's political prerogatives. As previously reported by the Select Subcommittee, Dr. Alexander, who was recruited by the Trump Administration in April 2020, was an outspoken advocate within the White House for policies that would allow the virus to spread widely among many Americans. Dr. Alexander also engaged in a persistent pattern of overruling and bullying scientists who advocated public health policies that went again the Trump Administration's perceived political interests.[52]

In December 2020, the Select Subcommittee detailed two separate instances first reported in the press that September in which Mr. Caputo bullied and threatened to retaliate against CDC personnel after they provided truthful information to the press without Mr. Caputo's permission.[53] In one instance, a *CNN* reporter had written to Mr. Caputo in June, asking whether "Operation Warp Speed is working on a vaccine education campaign." After Mr. Caputo refused to confirm the story, the reporter followed up, noting that a career CDC official had referred her to Mr. Caputo and had indicated that Mr. Caputo was "spearheading" the campaign. Mr. Caputo rebuked the career official for providing the information to *CNN*, writing: "In what world did you think it was your job to announce an Administration public service announcement to CNN?" He later followed up, stating, "[w]e will discuss this on a teleconference tomorrow. I want your HR representative in attendance." Mr. Caputo added Dr. Redfield to the exchange, writing, "I'm adding Dr Redfield back in this email exchange. Do not remove him again."[54] Ms. Galatas characterized Mr. Caputo's reaction as "threatening and unnecessary and not helpful," saying "we all had enough going on at the time, so I just didn't think that this was productive or helpful."[55]

Mr. Caputo also attempted to retaliate after a senior CDC scientist was interviewed by *NPR* about the Trump Administration's decision to strip CDC of its longstanding role in collecting hospital data, which experts warned could cause researchers, reporters, and the public to lose access to crucial data needed to combat the pandemic.[56] When Mr. Caputo learned the interview had occurred without his permission, he demanded to know the name of the CDC press officer who arranged it, warning CDC's senior staff: "If you disobey my directions, you will be held accountable." Following Mr. Caputo's outburst, Ms. Galatas informed Mr. Caputo that the incident was a mistake and that CDC was planning to issue the employee a "formal letter of reprimand." Mr. Caputo was unappeased, demanding an immediate meeting with the CDC employee, suggesting that that if he "wants an HR or union representative . . . that's preferable."[57] In an email previously released by the Select Subcommittee, Ms. Galatas wrote to HHS's Deputy Chief Counsel about Mr. Caputo's conduct following these two incidents, describing it as "a pattern of hostile and threatening behavior directed at me, Michelle [Bonds, Director of CDC's Division of Public Affairs], and communication staff at CDC."[58] During a transcribed interview, Ms. Galatas affirmed this sentiment to Select Subcommittee staff, saying that Mr. Caputo was "very threatening," that he exhibited "bully-ish behavior," and that he "definitely wanted us [CDC communications personnel] to feel threatened."[59]

Mr. Caputo also closely monitored the information career CDC scientists provided to the public and expressed his displeasure when they failed to stay on the message that the Trump Administration wanted them to convey. For example, on June 12, 2020, Dr. Butler led a CDC telebriefing—ending the agency's three-month period of silence—during which he acknowledged that it may be necessary to reinstate mitigation measures, saying: "if cases begin to go up again, and particularly if they go up dramatically, it's important to recognize that more intensive mitigation efforts such as what were implemented in March may be needed again."[60] During his transcribed interview, Dr. Butler stated that he learned after the telebriefing that Mr. Caputo was "very displeased by some of my responses." Although he did not speak directly to Mr. Caputo, Dr. Butler heard "secondhand" that Mr. Caputo believed that he "was not sticking to the talking points" and that he was "being too alarming about the state of the pandemic." Dr. Butler told the Select Subcommittee that he believed the information he shared at the telebriefing "was correct and, ultimately, is what helped limit the second wave," but he was only allowed to participate in one additional telebriefing and then "was not really asked back to do telebriefings."[61] Dr. Butler described the effect Mr. Caputo, and his office, had on CDC officials, saying:

> [S]ome people [at CDC] were intimidated . . . some of the behavior was just inexplicable. It was a little frustrating, though, because it's a distraction. It slows down the communication. And I think it really draws away from the important public health messages.[62]

Dr. Alexander similarly attacked CDC scientists who provided truthful information to the public when he felt that they contradicted Trump Administration talking points. In a new email obtained by the Select Subcommittee, Dr. Alexander wrote to Mr. Caputo and other Trump Administration political appointees about a forthcoming CDC scientific report about coronavirus risks to children, which he claimed was "garbage" and an attempt "to hurt the public and the administration." Dr. Alexander advocated for CDC officials to be fired, saying "he [Dr. Redfield] gots [sic] to start firing people in large numbers there! This agency is working against the President daily!"[63] In another email—which was previously detailed by the Select Subcommittee in a December 16, 2020, staff memorandum—Dr. Alexander called Dr. Schuchat "duplicitous" and accused her of lying about coronavirus risks after she provided accurate information about the worsening state of the coronavirus pandemic in an interview in late June 2020.[64] A new document shows that Mr. Caputo forwarded Dr. Alexander's incendiary attacks against Dr. Schuchat to Dr. Redfield and two other political appointees. When Dr. Alexander told Mr. Caputo "You must think I am a nut how I wrote here," Mr. Caputo responded that his email "Makes sense actually."[65]

In other instances, ASPA officials sought to insert their own messaging into CDC communications, including Dr. Redfield's public talking points. On May 8, 2020, a CDC Press

Officer emailed career ASPA staff seeking clearance for Dr. Redfield to participate in an interview about the effects of the pandemic on childhood vaccinations. The email indicated that Dr. Redfield "would strongly like to participate in this interview" and included a list of "cleared talking points." The email was then forwarded to Dr. Alexander who replied, seeking to insert his own messaging into Dr. Redfield's talking points and saying:[66]

> The key is to highlight that we are all not equally at risk and children [are] at minimal risk based on how the virus has been characterized thus far . . . . [W]e need to communicate that we are all not at equal risk. In US, CDC data suggests children 0-19 years old have risk of 0%.

Ms. Galatas told the Select Subcommittee that it was "unusual to have someone who was trying to do what looked like scientific clearance in the comms chain." She expressed her belief that "Paul Alexander and others from ASPA [were] trying to influence what the CDC director was saying" and said, "that's just not how we operate within CDC or with ASPA traditionally."[67] It is not clear whether Dr. Redfield used the talking points.

In June 2020, the White House installed two additional political appointees at CDC—Nina Witkofsky, who was initially appointed as a Senior Communications Advisor to Dr. Redfield and later assumed the role of Acting Chief of Staff, and Trey Moeller, who served as Ms. Witkofsky's deputy—neither of whom possessed prior public health experience. Ms. Witkofsky, who had previously volunteered at a CDC event for President Trump and worked for past Republican presidents, told the Select Subcommittee during a transcribed interview that she was approached to fill the positions at CDC by either the HHS White House Liaison or the White House Office of Presidential Personnel.[68]

Ms. Galatas recounted to the Select Subcommittee that Ms. Witkofsky told CDC communications staff shortly after she joined the agency that "she was in charge of CDC comms." According to Ms. Galatas, CDC's communications "would have been my purview as the then acting communications director for the agency," and that Ms. Witkofsky's installment "narrowed" her responsibilities. She explained that Ms. Witkofsky took over:

All media clearance, all support to the CDC director for his comms. And pretty much all of the response communications. So just everything that we were doing at the time related to the response. She kind of took over the communication leadership of that effort.[69]

Ms. Galatas stated that, based on her 20 years of experience at CDC, it was "unusual" for someone without any experience in public health to take over all communications for the agency and that "the overall impact" of Ms. Witkofsky's newfound control over CDC communications "slowed a lot of things down."[70] Despite her lack of public health background, Ms. Witkofsky participated in daily ASPA calls with Mr. Caputo, which no other CDC officials attended, attended meetings with public health officials, and was involved in policy discussions at CDC.[71] Ms. Witkofsky served as a key ally for ASPA within CDC—helping to funnel internal agency information to Mr. Caputo and his deputies and strategizing to rebut CDC findings perceived to be disadvantageous to the Trump Administration.[72]

E. Trump Administration Officials Sought to Downplay Risks Posed by the Coronavirus to Help President Trump's Perceived Political Interests

Instead of focusing on sharing truthful information about the pandemic to the American people, Trump Administration officials sought to coopt messaging from the nation's public health agencies to bolster President Trump's political prospects. As part of this effort, Dr. Alexander repeatedly attempted to alter CDC and HHS press materials to promote positive news, downplay coronavirus risks, and place responsibility on Democrats and past administrations—in an apparent attempt to redirect blame away from the Trump Administration for its poor handling of the coronavirus pandemic.

A new email obtained by the Select Subcommittee reveals that on May 8, 2020, Dr. Alexander sought to make changes to a CDC press statement that referenced the disproportionate impact of the coronavirus pandemic on people of color to stress that health disparities were "endemic and long-standing." He explained: "I will always know the words to use or discussion to blend the medicine with the politics…saying the economic issues are longstanding and endemic points to the past administrations and democratic govn [sic][.]"[73]

The next day, Dr. Alexander provided comments on CDC talking points about a new report on the impact of the pandemic on childhood immunizations. In a new email obtained by the Select Subcommittee, he told a CDC official that "the key message to slip in here is that the risk of death is 0%" for people 19 years old and younger from the coronavirus.[74] Dr. Alexander forwarded this response to Mr. Caputo, saying: "this is how I am supporting the messaging. . . . Any way to help you and showcase your work for this great President."[75]

In a May 19, 2020, email previously released by the Select Subcommittee, HHS senior advisor Brad Traverse wrote to Dr. Alexander, Mr. Caputo, and other HHS staff that he was concerned that a press article on coronavirus risk could be touted "as a reason not to open up America in red states." In response, Dr. Alexander suggested downplaying coronavirus risks by comparing the virus to the seasonal flu, writing "we can explain it this way: The risk in US or even globally of persons 60 years and less is less than seasonal influenza, the data shows this."[76]

On May 28, 2020, an official from ASPA circulated a draft CDC statement on the coronavirus death toll reaching 100,000 in the United States. In a new email obtained by the Select Subcommittee, Dr. Alexander responded with comments that he said were designed to make the statement "more positive." He explained that he deleted a reference to "100,000" lives lost in the title and removed other language calling the death toll "a sobering development and a heart-breaking reminder of the horrible toll of this unprecedented pandemic" because he thought it was too "heavy." CDC did not ultimately make the changes proposed by Dr. Alexander.[77]

As detailed in a December 16, 2020, staff report, Dr. Alexander wrote to officials at CDC and HHS on May 30, 2020, with comments on a CDC press statement regarding coronavirus hospitalization rates by race and ethnicity. He stated:[78]

Here is the issue: if the communication is left with just the statement that minoring [sic] groups are at higher risk then on its face this is very accurate, however, in this election cycle that is the kind of statement coming from CDC that the media and Democrat [sic] antagonists will use against the president. . . . each time we talk about these deaths we need to tell the nation why these deaths happened. This was due to decades of democrat [sic] neglect[.]

On June 15, 2020, Dr. Alexander urged HHS staff to release more "positive statements" supporting the Administration's pandemic response, saying that public health officials should "state that this President, this govn [sic], this Secretary, has done a good job and it is getting better. And we will be alright."[79]

Five days later, on June 20, 2020, Mr. Caputo responded to a draft CDC statement regarding extending the ban on passenger cruise ship travel asking: "Is this press release supposed to frighten readers?" Dr. Alexander replied that he made revisions to the draft statement and "toned it down," noting "such a piece needs to not frighten, but inform and constantly showcase the good work and hope etc."[80]

Following an alarming surge in cases in June 2020, Dr. Alexander discussed the "key message" to communicate to the public regarding the pandemic in a June 24 email. He wrote: "If we test more we will find more…but are the new cases problematic??? That's the key…" Dr. Alexander added: "We need also to tout the good stories as we know of elderly with serious conditions who get it and survive…this is key to tell…"[81]

II. The Trump White House Flagrantly Interfered in CDC's Coronavirus Guidance, Compromising Multiple Public Health Recommendations

The Trump White House interfered in the process for drafting, clearing, and issuing CDC coronavirus guidance during the early months of the pandemic.[82] White House officials without any background in infectious diseases overruled CDC scientists to weaken the public health recommendations in several coronavirus guidance documents—burying and obscuring the prevailing best practices while prioritizing the White House's favored interests.

A. The Trump White House Asserted Control over CDC's Coronavirus Guidance

As the pandemic took hold in the United States, the Trump White House began asserting control over CDC's guidance process. In prior emergencies, CDC spearheaded an interagency process to develop public health guidance that was clearly articulated and supported by the best available data.[83] But according to Dr. Schuchat, under the Trump Administration "the kinds of things that needed to have the view of outside the agency at HHS or the White House or OMB, the list expanded[.]"[84] Dr. Schuchat explained: "There was a lot of reluctance for almost anything to leave the agency."[85]

CDC's coronavirus guidance received particular scrutiny from officials at Office of Management and Budget (OMB), led by OMB Director Russell Vought. Documents previously released by the Select Subcommittee show that Mr. Vought, Office of Information and Regulatory Affairs (OIRA) Administrator Paul Ray, and other senior OMB officials coordinated with multiple White House officials—including Mr. Short and Counselor to the President Kellyanne Conway—in an effort to weaken CDC's coronavirus guidance and make it more politically palatable.[86] In her transcribed interview, Dr. Schuchat explained this "very unusual process" for clearing CDC's coronavirus guidance during the Trump Administration:

> [I]n this response was—there was kind of this vicious cycle that the White House task force would ask for something, we would draft it. OMB would say, why are you doing this? Then we would go back to the White House task force and then they would come back to us. Things were just spinning around in that world.[87]

Dr. Redfield told the Select Subcommittee that OMB officials effectively wielded veto power over his agency's coronavirus guidance, stating "we didn't get the approval usually to issue the guidance until OMB gave it a thumb's up."[88] In discussing OMB's involvement in CDC's guidance, Dr. Redfield said "onerous would be a polite word" for describing this process.[89] In a transcribed interview with the Select Subcommittee, White House Coronavirus Response Coordinator Dr. Deborah Birx explained that the White House clearance process that ran through OMB and OIRA took place outside of the White House Coronavirus Task Force, stating, "I have no understanding of that OIRA process and who was on that process and what guidance the CDC and changes they received out of that process, because that was parallel to the task force."[90]

A new email shows that Trump Administration officials went to OMB to seek changes to CDC guidance in an effort to deemphasize the importance of asymptomatic testing in high-risk congregate facilities. On June 17, 2020, a DHS official circulated updated CDC testing guidance that recommended deploying an asymptomatic testing program to prevent outbreaks in "special settings," including correctional and detention facilities.[91] Ken Cuccinelli, the DHS Senior Official Performing the Duties of the Deputy Secretary, forwarded the recommendation to Mr. Ray, saying: "Please advise." Mr. Ray told Mr. Vought that the guidance "is pretty bad," after which Mr. Vought raised the guidance directly with White House Chief of Staff Mark Meadows, writing: "It never ends."[92] When CDC released updated testing guidance for special settings two weeks later, all references to correctional or detention facilities had been removed, and the guidance instead advised special settings to contact their state or local health departments if they sought guidance on setting up asymptomatic testing programs.[93]

CDC's role in drafting and leading on coronavirus guidance was increasingly marginalized throughout 2020. Dr. Schuchat told the Select Subcommittee that "there was a point where we were not really asked to develop guidance" any longer, but instead "were asked to review guidance somebody else might have written and make sure this is okay. Sometimes our comments were taken and sometimes they weren't."[94] As CDC was further sidelined, Dr. Schuchat said that Kyle McGowan, CDC's Chief of Staff, "was trying to help keep things moving and negotiate" the content of guidance documents with White House officials.[95] Mr. McGowan and CDC Deputy Chief of Staff Amanda Campbell said that officials outside of CDC who disagreed with the recommendations in draft CDC guidance at times sought to circumvent the interagency process altogether and "take comments directly to Dr. Redfield."[96]

When asked about CDC's process for developing coronavirus guidance during the first year of the pandemic, Dr. Redfield acknowledged that it "got complicated" and commented that the process gave him "PTSD."[97] According to Dr. Schuchat, the process used to shape CDC's coronavirus guidance under the Trump Administration was "highly unusual."[98]

B. Trump White House Officials "Compromised" Multiple Coronavirus Guidance Documents

The Trump White House's involvement in CDC's coronavirus guidance process led to the issuance of multiple guidance documents that were coopted by political calculations and did not reflect the prevailing public health best practices.[99] During his transcribed interview, Dr. Redfield acknowledged that Trump Administration officials succeeded in undermining CDC's coronavirus guidance on multiple occasions, stating: "There was a couple of times where it was compromised."[100] Dr. Schuchat similarly told the Select Subcommittee that an internal review she conducted in the first months of 2021 found that multiple coronavirus guidance documents posted on CDC's website during the Trump Administration were not primarily authored by CDC.[101]

The Select Subcommittee's investigation has found that senior Trump Administration officials sought to interfere with—and in multiple instances succeeded in altering—the public health recommendations in multiple CDC coronavirus guidance documents, including:[102]

- Opening Up America Again, released on April 16, 2020. Dr. Schuchat confirmed in her transcribed interview that CDC removed this guidance document from its website in February 2021 "because it was not primarily drafted by us."[103]

- Memorandum on Strategies to Reduce COVID-19 Transmission at the Smithfield Foods Sioux Falls Pork Plant, dated April 22, 2020. Trump Administration officials coordinated with Smithfield Foods executives to water down CDC's recommendations to the meatpacking company to address a large-scale coronavirus outbreak at one of its plants.[104]

- Considerations for Restaurants and Bars, published in May 2020.[105] Trump White House officials successfully pressed CDC to remove a clear definition of "social distancing" from its decision tree for industry and to instead use an "ambiguous" standard.[106]

- Interim Guidance for Faith Communities, published on May 23, 2020.[107] The Trump White House directed CDC to replace its guidance with a weaker version drafted by White House officials who lacked any public health expertise.[108]

- Considerations for Election Polling Locations and Voters, published on June 22, 2020.[109] Dr. Schuchat said she found it "surprising" that the mail-in voting recommendation was removed from the guidance because this change was "counter to commonsense at that point."[110]

- The Importance of Reopening of America's Schools this Fall, published on July 23, 2020. Dr. Schuchat told the Select Subcommittee that CDC "was handed this essentially to post and had not drafted it," confirming it was developed and finalized outside of CDC.[111]

- Overview of Testing for SARS-CoV-2 (COVID-19), published on August 24, 2020.[112] Trump Administration officials, including Special Advisor to the President Dr. Scott Atlas, successfully weakened CDC's testing guidance to reduce the amount of testing conducted, months before any vaccines were authorized.

This pervasive interference in CDC's guidance not only sowed confusion about public health best practices, it resulted in published guidance that did not fully reflect leading experts' recommendations on how Americans could best protect themselves and their families from the coronavirus.

1.   *The Trump White House Directed CDC to Weaken Guidance for Faith Communities, Resulting in Guidance that CDC Experts Feared Would Cause Americans to "Get Sick and Perhaps Die"*

In April 2020, CDC drafted guidance for faith communities and sent a draft to the White House for clearance.[113] Dr. Butler, one of the public health experts involved in drafting these guidelines, said that CDC sought "to use the science [to] develop guidelines that can protect people to be able to worship in the way that's consistent with their faith and their tradition." Yet many of the public health recommendations crafted by CDC's subject matter experts were met with swift condemnation by the Trump White House.[114] The Select Subcommittee's investigation has uncovered that Trump Administration officials intervened to prevent CDC from initially releasing guidance for faith communities, and then ordered the agency to replace its guidance with a watered-down version drafted by the White House.

On April 18, 2020, White House officials raised their concerns about CDC's draft guidance for faith communities in internal emails. Denzel McGuire, an Associate Director at OMB, sent the draft directly to Mr. Vought, warning: "You are not going to like what they said about communion, I sure didn't."[115] White House officials thereafter made edits to CDC's draft guidance and sent their revised draft back to CDC.[116] Days later, Dr. Redfield sent White House officials the interim guidance for various settings, including guidance for communities of faith that did not fully reflect the edits previously provided by the White House.[117] In a document previously released by the Select Subcommittee, Jennie Lichter, a lawyer serving as Deputy Director of the Domestic Policy Council,[118] proposed that the White House override CDC's decision not to accept the White House's preferred edits:

> **From:** "Lichter, Jennie B. EOP/WHO" ◄ ████████████████████
> **Date:** April 25, 2020 at 9:02:46 AM EDT
> **To:** "Hirsch, Quinn N. EOP/OMB" ◄ ████████████████████
> **Cc:** "Higgins, Cortney J. EOP/OMB" ◄ ████████████████ "Grogan, Joseph J.
> EOP/WHO" ◄ ████████████████ "Ray, Paul J. EOP/OMB"
> ◄ ████████████
> **Subject:** RE: FLASH CLEARANCE by 9 PM TONIGHT (4/24): CDC Meatpacking & Reopening Guidance
>
> BUT what I'd prefer to do is resubmit the combined edits you produced for the last round (Weds evening edit) to CDC as my submission on the faith section. CDC appears to have accepted virtually none of the comments or edits submitted by me, DOJ, or anyone else on this very sensitive section last time, and that is unacceptable.
>
> sensitive section last time, and that is unacceptable.
>
> Thanks,
> Jennie

White House Domestic Policy Council Director Joe Grogan advocated that the White House circumvent CDC altogether: "Actually I am not sure these should go back to cdc. I think we should make the edits and then a small group of principals finalize." Mr. Vought likewise replied: "Agreed. They didn't take any of my edits either."[119]

The next day, Mr. Ray circulated updated drafts of the reopening guidance to senior White House officials. The email, which was previously released by the Select Subcommittee, attached the Trump White House's version of the faith communities guidance with recommendations that were not supported by CDC's experts:[120]

From: Ray, Paul J. EOP/OMB ███████████████
Sent: Sunday, April 26, 2020 6:44 PM
To: Birx, Deborah L. EOP/NSC ███████████████ Grogan, Joseph J. EOP/WHO
███████████████ Bonner, Maria K. EOP/WHO
███████████████ ; Lichter, Jennie B. EOP/WHO
███████████████ ; Vought, Russell T. EOP/OMB
███████████████ Kan, Derek T. EOP/OMB ███████████████
Short, Marc T. EOP/OVP ███████████████ ; Troye, Olivia EOP/NSC

Subject: Fwd: guidance and decision trees

Hi all—at request of Joe and Russ, I'm attaching here for your review and edits the current drafts of the re-opening guidance and decision trees. These drafts are the product of the agency resolution processes held over the weekend (with the exception of the faith-based guidance; I am circulating the EOP-preferred version of that guidance, with which CDC has maintained disagreement).

Sent from my iPhone

Around the same time, White House officials became aware of existing guidance posted on CDC's website that was designed to assist faith community leaders to "prevent the transmission of COVID-19 within their facilities and communities."[121] On April 28, 2020, Ms. Miller, Vice President Pence's Press Secretary, sent senior OMB officials a link to this guidance, asking: "We're [sic] you aware of this?" Mr. Vought replied that "This looks really old," while another OMB official explained that it was "from late March," "not vetted through the WH," and "was heavy handed." The OMB official added Mr. Short to the email to alert him about the guidance.[122]

Two days later, HHS disseminated a link to this guidance to Administration officials as part of a broader update on the coronavirus response. Ms. Lichter forwarded the update to Mr. Grogan, Mr. Ray, and other senior White House officials, writing:

> I am dying right now—HHS blasted out this email touting "new webpages with reopening information and resources" for a bunch of sectors, including the faith community—so I ask myself, hmm, have we approved new reopening resources for all of these groups? Turns out no, the link for faith community (for example) goes to this page: [hyperlink] which, despite being dated April 30, takes you to the bad old CDC guidance that they posted in March without asking us [hyperlink] and that says consider modifying or suspending communion.[123]

CDC released reopening guidance documents for specific settings, including mass transit, schools, and workplaces, on May 14, 2020—but omitted any guidance for faith communities.[124]

An internal CDC email obtained by the Select Subcommittee documented that the agency was "instructed" to release its reopening guidance "in pieces with the faith-based guidance stripped out."[125] In his transcribed interview, Dr. Butler acknowledged that the faith communities guidance suffered the "longest delay" of all CDC coronavirus guidance.[126]

A week after CDC released its other reopening guidance, Jennifer Dickey, Deputy Associate Attorney General at the Department of Justice (DOJ), reached out to Ms. Lichter and May Davis, Associate White House Counsel, on May 21, 2020, inquiring about CDC's existing guidance for faith leaders. In a document previously released by the Select Subcommittee, Ms. Dickey noted that "some folks here [are] raising concerns about the fact that the 'interim' CDC guidance on houses of worship is still online," and asked if there was "any plan for HHS to take that down/be replaced?" Ms. Davis forwarded this message to senior OMB officials, "[f]lagging that the problematic guidance is still online" and explaining that she "tried to make the changes in the attached (on top of Kellyanne edits) to get over to OIRA today"—an apparent reference to Ms. Conway.[127] Ms. Davis noted that, with her edits, the revised version of the guidance "removes all of the tele-church suggestions, though personally I will say that if I was old and vulnerable (I do feel old and vulnerable), drive through services would sound welcome."[128]

Later that day, an aide to Ms. Conway sent Mr. McGowan at CDC a revised version of the faith communities guidance.[129] President Trump announced during an event at an automobile manufacturing facility that afternoon that he had spoken to CDC and the public was "going to see something come out very soon about opening up our churches."[130] An email previously released by the Select Subcommittee shows that Mr. McGowan sent a group of senior White House officials a further revised draft of the guidance that evening, which Ms. Conway promptly forwarded to Mr. Ray, who replied:

From: Conway, Kellyanne E. EOP/WHO
Sent: Friday, May 22, 2020 1:10 AM
To: Ray, Paul J. EOP/OMB
Cc: Lyons, Derek S. EOP/WHO   Philbin, Patrick F. EOP/WHO
                              Joannou, Tom W. EOP/WHO
                              Troye, Olivia EOP/NSC   Vought,
Russell T. EOP/OMB   Lichter, Jennie B. EOP/WHO

Subject: Re: Faith Guidance

Paul - Thanks for adding our colleagues who have been central to this effort. Thanks, also, for

> The new CDC draft includes a significant amount of new content, much of which seems to raise religious liberty concerns. In the attached, I have proposed several passages for deletion to address those concerns (as well as a few other necessary edits). If these edits are acceptable to you all, we could tell CDC, as early in the morning as possible, that they are free to publish contingent on striking the offensive passages.

Thank you, Kellyanne. Adding Russ, Jennie, and Olivia as well. The new CDC draft includes a significant amount of new content, much of which seems to raise religious liberty concerns. In the attached, I have proposed several passages for deletion to address those concerns (as well as a few other necessary edits). If these edits are acceptable to you all, we could tell CDC, as early in the morning as possible, that they are free to publish contingent on striking the offensive passages.

PREDECISIONAL DELIBERATIVE

Paul J. Ray
Administrator
Office of Information and Regulatory Affairs
Office of Management and Budget

Ms. Conway thanked Mr. Ray for his efforts to hold firm on the guidance, and Ms. Lichter sent an additional "few comments to Paul's" revised draft.[131]

From: Conway, Kellyanne E. EOP/WHO ██████████████

Sent: Friday, May 22, 2020 1:10 AM

To: Ray, Paul J. EOP/OMB ████████████████████

Cc: Lyons, Derek S. EOP/WHO ██████████████ Philbin, Patrick F. EOP/WHO ██████████████████ Joannou, Tom W. EOP/WHO ███████████████ Troye, Olivia EOP/NSC ██████████████████; Vought, Russell T. EOP/OMB ██████████████████ Lichter, Jennie B. EOP/WHO ███████████████

Subject: Re: Faith Guidance

Paul - Thanks for adding our colleagues who have been central to this effort. Thanks, also, for holding firm against the newest round of mission creep.

Kellyanne Conway
Counselor to the President
Executive Office of the President
Office: ███████████

The following morning, in a document previously released by the Select Subcommittee, Mr. Ray asked the White House to send any other edits to the draft guidance by 10 a.m., "[i]n view of what I understand to be potential POTUS activity on this[.]" Ms. Conway offered her support for the White House's changes, replying: "All set here as well."[132] That afternoon, President Trump announced: "At my direction, the Centers for Disease Control and Prevention is issuing guidance for communities of faith." He threatened to "override" state leaders if they did not reopen churches and other places of worship "right now."[133]

The CDC subject matter experts developing coronavirus guidance received little advanced notice from the White House that President Trump would be issuing these directives. In his transcribed interview, Dr. Butler—who was serving as CDC's Incident Manager for the coronavirus response at the time—told the Select Subcommittee that he and his team "were not aware that the President would be announcing that the guidelines had been posted," which "created a tight timeline to get it posted." When asked whether he would have recommended that all houses of worship open "right now," as President Trump demanded, Dr. Butler replied: "I wouldn't have, no." Dr. Butler said that the President's directive at that time "gives me a great deal of pause."[134]

Hours after President Trump's press conference ended, CDC posted the "Interim Guidance for Communities of Faith" to its website.[135] However, the version that CDC posted was not the version that contained the Trump White House's preferred recommendations— prompting the White House and Dr. Redfield to swiftly order Dr. Butler's team to pull down its guidance and replace it with the White House's version.[136] During his transcribed interview,

Dr. Butler recalled "being contacted by the White House" on the evening of Saturday, May 23, 2020, and speaking with a staffer in the Office of the Vice President, as well as with Dr. Redfield and Mr. McGowan. Dr. Butler explained that he was informed that CDC's guidance "had not been fully cleared." He said the call made him feel "confused" and gave him "concern," but that he and his team moved quickly that night "to replace the version that was posted with the cleared version."[137] Dr. Redfield told the Select Subcommittee that CDC initially posted an "incorrect version" of the guidance by mistake.[138] According to Dr. Schuchat, the Trump White House prevented CDC from releasing the version of the guidance supported by the agency's experts: "we were asked to develop the faith-based guidance, and not able to release it based on concerns from those, OMB, OIRA, intergovernmental reviews."[139]

A new email obtained by the Select Subcommittee shows that Olivia Troye, an adviser to Vice President Pence, contacted Ms. Conway, Ms. Lichter, Mr. Short, Mr. Vought, and other White House officials the night of May 23, 2020, informing them:

> The correct guidance is up on the CDC website now. Dr. Redfield worked with his team this evening to rectify this situation. I've been on the phone with his team this evening as well as a few others internally within the WH. This is now resolved.[140]

Dr. Redfield acknowledged in his transcribed interview that the faith communities guidance "went through just way too many iterations, took way too long to get posted, way too many disagreements" and "was one of the most contentious guidance that I had to be involved with, period."[141]

After complying with the White House's order, Dr. Butler and his team composed a timeline of events leading up to the White House's directive to remove and replace the faith communities guidance and conducted a review to "cross-check the two versions to see what were the differences" between the version CDC initially posted and the final version demanded by the White House.[142] These differences were documented in an internal email obtained by the Select Subcommittee in which Dr. Butler outlined a series of changes that the White House made— including removing references to face coverings, eliminating suggestions for virtual services, and cutting recommendations to consider reducing lines and limiting the use of choirs. In the email, Dr. Butler told his team, "as someone who has been speaking with churches and pastors on this (and as someone who goes to church), I am not sure is [sic] see a public health reason to take down and replace." Dr. Butler further detailed how the White House's changes were divorced from any clear public health objective:

> The version we had to post tonight does not have answers to a number of the questions that we have been asked by the faith community and lacks a number of recommendations for other settings to support reopening as safely as possible.[143]

After comparing the two versions, Dr. Butler concluded that the White House's version of the guidance "is not good public health" and told his team:[144]

From:	Butler, Jay C. (CDC/DDID/OD)
To:	McQuiston, Jennifer H. (CDC/DDID/NCEZID/DHCPP)
Cc:	Fitter, David L. (CDC/DDPHSIS/CGH/GID); Eisenberg, Emily (CDC/DDID/NCIRD/ID)
Subject:	Re: Faith-based guidance and COVID-19: A history
Date:	Sunday, May 24, 2020 7:46:38 AM

Thank you, Jenni—I appreciate the additional information and so much hard work and midnight oil that went into developing a very good public health document under incredible time pressure, and in getting the original post up Friday with very little notice. I also appreciate everyone's agile responsiveness in getting the WH version up ASAP last night, as we were directed to do. ██

This is not good public health—I am very troubled on this Sunday morning that there will be people who will get sick and perhaps die because of what we were forced to do. Our team has done the good work, only to have it compromised.

During his transcribed interview, Dr. Butler reiterated that the White House's version of the faith communities guidance "actually softened some of the recommendations in ways we found concerning," which he said "was really pretty demoralizing" for his team. He explained that multiple faith leaders had contacted CDC before guidance was issued to express "a lot of interest" in public health recommendations for their communities. Dr. Butler said CDC's version of the guidance "aligned with conversations that I had been having with pastors as something that would be acceptable." Based on his review of the White House's version, Dr. Butler said "[i]t seemed like the differences were not things that were going to be offensive" to faith communities, and that he has "yet to have anybody from any faith community tell me that I have offended them when I've talked about how respiratory particles are generated during speaking, shouting, or singing."[145]

Reflecting on the "real struggle" he faced after receiving the directive from the White House to post its preferred guidance, Dr. Butler said that he "was doing a lot of soul searching about whether or not I should have agreed to even make the change in the document." Ultimately, he said: "I felt like what had been done was not good public health practice" and "will haunt me for some time."[146]

2. Trump OMB Officials Pressured CDC to Use an "Ambiguous" Social-Distancing Recommendation in Guidance for Restaurants and Bars

Evidence obtained by the Select Subcommittee shows that Trump White House officials pressured CDC to change its guidance for restaurants and bars to provide less direct recommendations for how to keep patrons and employees safe.[147] According to Dr. Butler, by the spring of 2020, CDC had accumulated "evidence of significant community transmission" in bars and restaurants, and began drafting guidance designed to mitigate transmission in these settings.[148] In a written submission to the Select Subcommittee, Mr. McGowan and Ms. Campbell detailed that, as CDC was drafting this guidance, "OMB informed CDC that the inclusion of social distancing in the guidance was too prescriptive and would harm business" and "asked CDC to remove social distancing from the guidance." After CDC initially declined to do so, OMB "urged CDC to change the definition of social distancing from six feet to a more ambiguous standard."[149]

Mr. McGowan and Ms. Campbell informed the Select Subcommittee that CDC agreed to remove certain language from the guidance for restaurants and bars that provided a specific recommendation as to how far to keep customers apart. In its place, CDC inserted a hyperlink that would take a reader to a separate webpage where they could then find a more specific definition of social distancing. CDC's May 2020 decision tree for restaurants and bars advised the industry simply to "Encourage social distancing"—omitting any definition of the term in the guidance itself.[150]

When asked about these changes to the guidance for restaurants and bars, Dr. Henry Walke, who served as one of the Incident Managers for CDC's coronavirus response during the summer of 2020, told the Select Subcommittee that stripping out the more specific definition of social distancing from the guidance "doesn't make a lot of sense."[151]

3.   *The Trump White House Purposefully Weakened CDC's Testing Guidance to Curtail Testing*

As documented in a June 2022 staff report, evidence obtained by the Select Subcommittee reveals how Dr. Atlas set in motion significant changes to CDC's testing guidance that upended CDC's public health recommendations by minimizing the need for widespread testing and undercutting policies to mitigate the spread of the coronavirus. According to Dr. Redfield, "significant people" inside the Trump Administration made clear shortly after Dr. Atlas arrived at the White House in late July 2020 that "there needed to be some curtailment of the amount of testing that was done as relating to evaluating people that were exposed."[152]

Dr. Atlas's radical and politically charged views on testing were captured in an August 11, 2020, email from Dr. Birx obtained by the Select Subcommittee. In the email, Dr. Birx recounted a "very dangerous meeting in the OVAL yesterday" and detailed "Dr Atlas thoughts" on the pandemic, which indicated that President Trump had demanded changes to CDC's testing guidance: "Testing is very over rating [sic]—thus the source of the President's call for new testing guidance." Dr. Birx also indicated that Dr. Atlas was overtly mixing public health with politics by advocating the idea that "Case identification is bad for the President's reelection—testing should only be of the sick." Dr. Birx warned that, after the Oval Office meeting with Dr. Atlas, she believed "the President will be following his guidance now."[153]

Multiple former Trump Administration officials told the Select Subcommittee that Dr. Atlas spearheaded changes to CDC's testing guidance to stop recommending that all close contacts of individuals infected with the coronavirus get tested. Admiral Brett Giroir, the Trump Administration's "Testing Czar," recounted during a transcribed interview that the White House Coronavirus Task Force approved a draft of the weakened testing guidance that included a recommendation that all close contacts isolate for 14 days. Dr. Giroir said that he was surprised that the isolation recommendation was not included when the guidance was published on August 24, 2020.[154] According to Dr. Schuchat, the testing guidance was "another low point in confusion for our partners," as the revisions "didn't make sense to most of the public health community."[155]

Dr. Birx told the Select Subcommittee that she observed a "dramatic decline of the number of tests performed during the end of August and the beginning of September [2020]" following the release of this guidance, stating: "This document resulted in less testing and less—less aggressive testing of those without symptoms that I believed were the primary reason for the early community spread." In a September 16, email to senior White House officials, Dr. Birx noted that "this marks the third week with significant declines in testing and we cannot see the community spread that maybe [sic] happening," warning: "This requires immediate action by the CDC."[156]

In the face of the significant reduction in testing and a severe backlash from the public health community, CDC issued revised testing guidance on September 18, 2020, that aligned with the public health consensus that all close contacts of those infected with the coronavirus "need a test." Dr. Redfield told the Select Subcommittee that, after the revised guidance was published, Dr. Atlas "aggressively spoke to me in loud terms" and accused CDC of not having the White House Coronavirus Task Force's approval to change the guidance. Dr. Birx similarly said that other senior White House officials likewise objected to these science-based revisions.[157]

Based on his experience leading CDC amid the Trump White House's flagrant interference in the agency's coronavirus guidance, Dr. Redfield told the Select Subcommittee that he believes CDC needs structural reforms to better insulate the agency from these types of political pressures moving forward, calling for "greater independence with CDC, when it comes to making public health decisions."[158]

III.   **The Trump Administration Brazenly Interfered with CDC's Public Health Authorities**

Trump Administration officials repeatedly exploited and counteracted CDC's public health authorities to achieve political goals during the first year of the pandemic—instead of allowing CDC to use these authorities as intended to combat the coronavirus crisis. The Select Subcommittee's investigation has uncovered new evidence that Trump Administration officials usurped CDC's public health authorities to effectively close U.S. land borders to migrants seeking asylum under the guise of mitigating the spread of the coronavirus. Trump Administration officials also blocked CDC from exercising its public health powers to deploy one of the few effective tools then-available to mitigate the spread of the coronavirus and interfered with CDC's decision to extend a No Sail Order for the cruise line industry in the fall of 2020. This brazen interference with CDC's public health authorities resulted in policies and actions that, according to multiple CDC officials, did not appear to serve a compelling public health purpose.[159]

A. Trump Administration Officials Overruled Public Health Experts and Exploited CDC's Authorities to Close the Southern Border

On March 20, 2020, CDC issued an order pursuant to Title 42 of the Public Health Services Act requiring the expulsion of certain individuals seeking asylum protections at U.S. land borders under the purported justification that doing so was "necessary to protect the public health from an increase in the serious danger of the introduction of Coronavirus Disease 2019 (COVID-19)" (the Title 42 order).[160] The Select Subcommittee's investigation has found that the Title 42 order did not originate at CDC and that key CDC experts disagreed that there was a sufficient public health basis for the order.[161]

During a transcribed interview, Dr. Martin Cetron, Director of CDC's Division of Global Migration and Quarantine, told the Select Subcommittee that the idea for the Title 42 order "came from outside the CDC subject matter experts," and that "the proposed order was not drafted by me or my team" but was instead "handed to us."[162] Stephen Miller—a senior policy adviser to President Trump who was reportedly a driving force behind the Trump Administration's family separation policy and Muslim travel ban—was among those outside CDC who was involved in formulating the Title 42 order.[163] Although Dr. Redfield said in his transcribed interview that he was not aware of Mr. Miller's involvement in the Title 42 order,[164] Dr. Cetron told the Select Subcommittee that he recalled participating in calls "in which he [Mr. Miller] was speaking."[165]

Evidence obtained by the Select Subcommittee suggests that Trump Administration officials distorted the coronavirus-transmission risk posed by migrants at the time they advanced a public health justification for the Title 42 order. Dr. Cetron explained that the "argument about the risk of importing" coronavirus at the border "did not jibe" with the data and realities on the ground, particularly given that "there were hot spots in the U.S. that were much more powerfully overwhelming at the moment."[166] Dr. Cetron detailed how his team conducted an extensive analysis to assess the coronavirus risks migrants posed to the United States—which found that the sweeping scope of the Title 42 order was not justified on public health grounds:

> We looked at the rationale. We gathered data on the reported incidents of the disease in these populations. We scoured international available data. My team that works physically on the border, including the U.S.-Mexico unit and others with a lot of experience, we could not substantiate that the threat was, quote/unquote, being addressed by this. . . . [T]here were other very important sanitary measures and changes in capacities and cohorting and other tools that can and should be used and had been recommended many times in the past around this. And so that was our assessment.[167]

Consistent with this assessment, when asked about the justification for the Title 42 order, Dr. Schuchat told the Select Subcommittee: "the bulk of the evidence at that time did not support this policy proposal[.]"[168]

Dr. Cetron said that he and his team were concerned that "significant harms" could come from using the agency's public health authorities in this "unprecedented" manner.[169] Specifically, he "was concerned that there may be a motivation that was beyond the specific public health agenda" that was being advanced as the basis for the Title 42 order.[170] According to a press report, Dr. Cetron told a CDC colleague in March 2020 after receiving the proposed Title 42 order: "I will not be a part of this. It's just morally wrong to use a public authority that has never, ever, ever been used this way. It's to keep Hispanics out of the country. And it's wrong."[171] When asked about this statement in his transcribed interview, Dr. Cetron said that it was "consistent with some of the concerns that I had." Dr. Cetron explained that the order also risked creating "an inappropriate epidemic of stigma and misrepresentation of where the problem is," while "creating a false narrative" that the virus was contained outside the United States and Americans could "therefore avoid[] the kinds of things that we all need to be doing collectively to address the risk."[172]

Dr. Cetron said that he asked to "excuse" himself from working on the Title 42 order given the "potentially significant harms" implicated, after concluding that it was not justified under CDC's public health authorities.[173] He told the Select Subcommittee:

> I didn't feel that this approach met the responsibilities that we had taken on for using public health authorities appropriately, judiciously, most wisely, and with the least public health collateral damage. I thought some of these kinds of consequences that were not being realized would end up having greater both COVID consequences and other public health damaging consequences.[174]

Dr. Redfield elected to use CDC's public health authorities to execute the Title 42 order, although he acknowledged in his transcribed interview that "there were clearly people who had different points of view of how this authority should be used."[175] When asked if she knew why Dr. Redfield signed the Title 42 order given the lack of a clear public health rationale, Dr. Schuchat pointed to the intense political pressures that Dr. Redfield was subjected to as CDC Director, responding:[176]

Dr. Schuchat:	No. I imagine that Dr. Redfield was put in many impossible situations over the course of his position.
Majority Counsel:	By impossible situations, you mean the pressure from a political perspective?
Dr. Schuchat:	I would agree with that.

B. Trump Administration Officials Blocked CDC from Using Its Public Health Authorities to Deploy a Key Tool Ahead of the Fall and Winter 2020 Surge

Trump Administration officials prevented CDC from exercising its public health authorities to implement a mask requirement on public and commercial transportation within the United States. According to Dr. Cetron, CDC began working on the proposed order in July 2020, and the concept for a universal mask requirement on mass transportation enjoyed "fairly broad consensus" across CDC at that time. Dr. Cetron said that his team concluded that "the evidence was scientifically there" to support the proposed mask order and that CDC's internal modeling indicated that the order would be "significant in risk reduction" and a "potentially important tool in the tool kit that could make a big difference."[177] Dr. Schuchat similarly explained that the science at the time supported the proposed mask order, telling the Select Subcommittee: "If we were using the full strength of government to protect the nation, this was a reasonable move." Dr. Schuchat also underscored that the proposed mask order "was really desired on the part of industry." She said that "the transit industry was really interested in there being strong guidance" on masks, as were "lots of venues," both of which wanted "the federal government being more clear or strong about this."[178]

HHS leadership, including Secretary Azar and Dr. Redfield, expressed support for the proposed order, according to Dr. Cetron.[179] Dr. Birx said in her transcribed interview that she also supported the proposed mask order and recalled that Dr. Redfield was scheduled to present on the matter at a White House Coronavirus Task Force meeting, although she did not recall the presentation ever taking place.[180] A White House Coronavirus Task Force agenda obtained by the Select Subcommittee shows that Dr. Redfield and Department of Transportation Assistant Secretary Joel Szabat were scheduled to present on "Facial Coverings" at a July 31, 2020, Task Force meeting.[181]

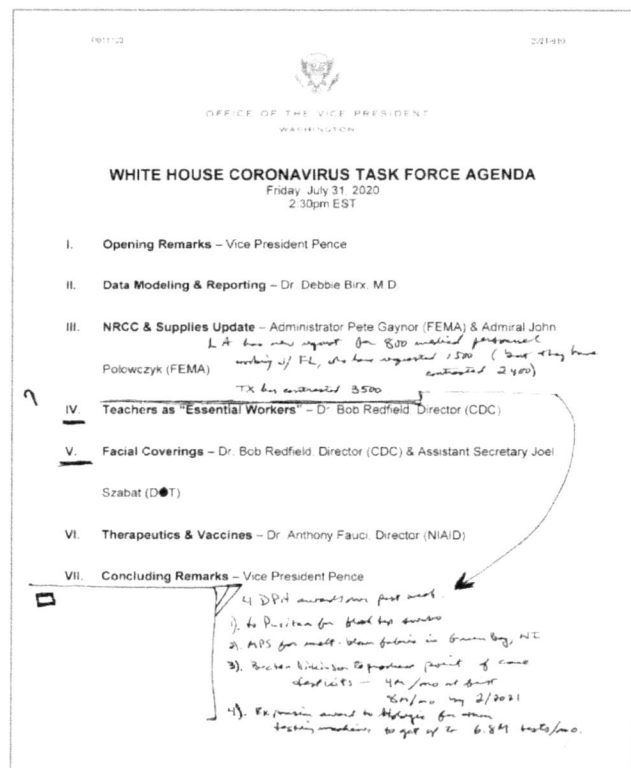

Despite widespread support for the proposed order among leading public health experts, Dr. Cetron said that CDC was told it "would not happen" and that "there would be no such use of federal authority for masking in a transportation corridor." He told the Select Subcommittee that he was not provided a specific reason why CDC was barred from issuing the proposed order despite the strong public health justification behind it. According to Dr. Cetron, the proposed mask order "was well within the scope of the federal public health authority that the CDC was given." Had CDC not been stymied by Trump Administration officials outside of HHS, Dr. Cetron believed the order "could have made a significant contribution" in the nation's efforts to save American lives from the coronavirus in 2020.[182]

C. CDC Extended Its No Sail Order Over the Trump White House's Objections

On March 14, 2020, CDC implemented a No Sail Order, suspending certain cruise ships from launching new voyages from U.S. ports after widespread coronavirus outbreaks onboard ships resulted in multiple deaths.[183] According to Dr. Schuchat, CDC was tracking "numerous outbreaks on cruise ships" around this time and determined "that it wasn't possible to make it safe for individuals, crew, or travelers to be on a cruise ship during this phase of transmission of the virus."[184] Dr. Cetron, whose division created a dedicated maritime unit to address coronavirus outbreaks on cruise ships, told the Select Subcommittee that a No Sail Order was necessary to "stop adding accelerant to the fire of these outbreaks" and to prevent more Americans from "getting severely ill or dying."[185] The March 14 order, however, excluded cruise operators that voluntarily suspended new operations from U.S. ports while the order was in effect, and did not cover ongoing ship operations and the tens of thousands of crew members actively onboard.[186]

In a newly released email sent on April 5, 2020, Dr. Cetron pressed CDC leadership to extend and expand the scope of the initial No Sail Order, citing ongoing outbreaks on multiple ships. Dr. Cetron warned Dr. Redfield and other senior CDC officials that the agency "urgently needed" to require all cruise ships "to cease operations" and "develop and implement an adequate response plan to COVID-19" as a condition to being present in any U.S. waters:[187]

Message	
From:	Cetron, Marty (CDC/DDID/NCEZID/DGMQ) [/O=EXCHANGELABS/OU=EXCHANGE ADMINISTRATIVE GROUP (FYDIBOHF23SPDLT)/CN=RECIPIENTS/CN=E961A00D121E4FE78303A319D7802398-CETRON, MAR]
Sent:	4/5/2020 5:03:05 PM
To:	Redfield, Robert R. (CDC/OD) ▓▓▓▓ McGowan, Robert (Kyle) (CDC/OD/OCS) ▓▓▓▓
CC:	Marty Cetron (CDC/OID/NCEZID) ▓▓▓▓ Misrahi, James J. (CDC/OCOO/OGC) ▓▓▓▓
	▓▓▓▓ (EHInternship) CDC, SUPEH (CDC) ▓▓▓▓
BCC:	Schuchat, Anne MD (CDC/OD)
Subject:	No Sail Order Cruise Ships_Extension_4-5-20 at 12PM.docx
Attachments:	No Sail Order Cruise Ships_Extension_4-5-20 at 12PM.docx
Flag:	Follow up

> Ongoing operations of overlast 3 weeks have revealed ongoing large and frequent COVID-19 outbreaks at sea involving multiple vessels and impacted countless passenger and crew; including many with COVID infections with severe disease requiring numerous medical evacuations of critical patients you and old and several deaths on board

- deaths on board
- Ongoing Cruise ship related COVID outbreaks continue to impose significant burdens on local, state, and federal

> Dozens of vessels are still at sea with active COVID infections on board are lingering nearby and heading toward

> A new NO Sail Order to cease operations with US Territorial waters is urgently needed to rectify this problem

> Within 7 days of signing, cruise ship operators must develop and implement an adequate response plan to COVID-19 that **does not post additional risk of COVID 19 spread nor burden federal, state, or local governments or the healthcare system as a condition of operating (being present) in any U.S. waters**

- emergency; or we rescind prior if PH circumstances warrant.
- Order does not prohibit humanitarian rescue on an emergency case-by-case basis.

MSC
Martin S. Cetron, MD, FIDSA, FASTMH
Director, Global Migration and Quarantine
CDC

In his transcribed interview, Dr. Cetron explained that a broader No Sail Order was necessary because his team obtained evidence suggesting that the industry's voluntary compliance was inadequate and "we needed a more uniform, consistent, clear set of instructions."[188]

White House Coronavirus Task Force agendas obtained by the Select Subcommittee show that the Task Force was scheduled to discuss a "No Sail Order Extension" on April 5 and April 7, 2020, respectively. According to the agendas, Acting DHS Secretary Chad Wolf was scheduled to lead the first presentation on the No Sail Order extension, and to co-lead the second presentation two days later with Dr. Redfield.[189]

OFFICE OF THE VICE PRESIDENT WASHINGTON	OFFICE OF THE VICE PRESIDENT WASHINGTON
WHITE HOUSE CORONAVIRUS TASK FORCE AGENDA Sunday, April 5, 2020 5:00pm EST	**WHITE HOUSE CORONAVIRUS TASK FORCE AGENDA** Tuesday, April 7, 2020 3:00pm EST
I. Opening Remarks – Vice President Pence	I. Opening Remarks – Vice President Pence
II. Data Modeling & Reporting Update – Dr. Debi Birx, M.D.	II. Data Modeling & Reporting Update – Dr. Debi Birx, M.D.
III. NRCC & Supplies Update – Administrator Pete Gaynor (FEMA) & Admiral John Polowczyk (FEMA)	○ Medical Work Streams
	○ Surgeon General Outreach & Data Disaggregation – Dr. Jerome Adams, US Surgeon General
○ Masks & Ventilators	III. NRCC & Supplies Update – Administrator Pete Gaynor (FEMA) & Admiral John Polowczyk (FEMA)
IV. Testing – Admiral Brett Giroir (HHS)	○ Ventilators
V. DOD & Veterans Affairs Support – Deputy Secretary David Norquist (DOD) & Secretary Robert Wilkie (VA)	IV. DOD & Veterans Affairs Support – Deputy Secretary David Norquist (DOD) & Secretary Robert Wilkie (VA)
VI. Cruise Ships – No Sail Order Extension – Acting Secretary Chad Wolf (DHS)	V. Testing – Admiral Brett Giroir (HHS)
VII. Concluding Remarks – Vice President Pence	○ Overall Strategy Update
	VI. Hazard Pay Recommendation – Russ Vought, Director (OMB)
	VII. DPA Request – Administrator Pete Gaynor (FEMA) & Pat Cipollone, Counsel to the President
	○ DO Designation for Zoll Supply Chain
	○ Temporary Final Rule – Allocation for Scarce or Threatened Materials
	○ Priority Related Orders on Health & Medical Resources
	VIII. Cruise Ship – No Sail Order Extension – Acting Secretary Chad Wolf (DHS) & Dr. Bob Redfield, Director (CDC)
	IX. Concluding Remarks – Vice President Pence

Dr. Cetron acknowledged in his transcribed interview that CDC encountered resistance during the interagency process that constrained the agency's ability to quickly issue an extended and expanded No Sail Order—suggesting that disagreements reportedly voiced by DHS officials were one of the sources for this delay.[190]

CDC ultimately announced on April 9, 2020, that it would be issuing an expanded No Sail Order effective April 15.[191] When asked about the delays he encountered, Dr. Cetron told the Select Subcommittee:

> I do think the delays or the frustration were some of the challenges that we had in getting to where we needed to in public health. I believe some of those things have cost lives, and I'm saddened by it.[192]

The No Sail Order was later modified and extended effective July 16 and September 30, after which it was set to expire on October 31, 2020.[193] Representatives of the cruise line industry and their allies, including Florida Governor Ron DeSantis, called on the Trump Administration to let the No Sail Order expire so cruise ships could resume operations.[194] Dr. Redfield noted that CDC also "had discussions with the industry" regarding the No Sail Order, including with members of a committee established and funded by several major cruise lines that was led by former Bush Administration HHS Secretary Michael Leavitt.[195] Handwritten notes on a White House Coronavirus Task Force agenda produced by the White House indicate that the Trump Administration was conducting "DeSantis outreach" in connection with the No Sail Order that summer.[196]

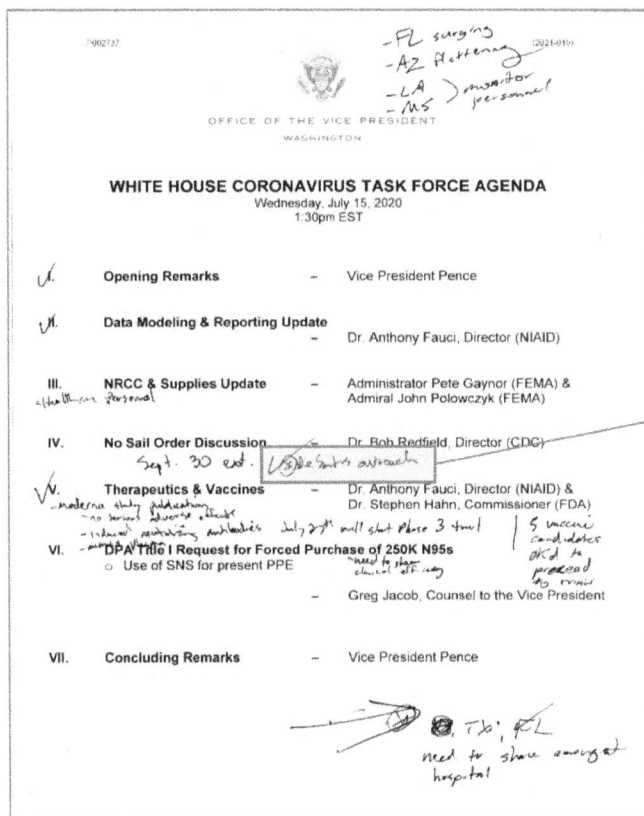

In his transcribed interview, Dr. Redfield said that he advocated extending the No Sail Order until March 2021, because he believed "human life was dependent on it."[197] Dr. Schuchat similarly told the Select Subcommittee that "it was inconceivable that everything was going to be fine" if the No Sail Order was allowed to expire at the end of October 2020.[198] Despite consensus from top CDC leadership on the need to extend the No Sail Order, Trump White House officials rejected this plan.[199] Dr. Redfield told the Select Subcommittee that "the Vice President made the decision" not to extend the No Sail Order through the winter, as Dr. Redfield had called for.[200]

Facing resistance to an extension, Dr. Redfield said he "came up with a new idea which was the Conditional Sail Order" that CDC ultimately issued on October 30, 2020.[201] Dr. Redfield explained that the industry-sponsored committee led by former Secretary Leavitt "came up with a great document" that specified steps industry would take before resuming operations, "[a]nd that's what led me to say, that sounds good, let's put a Conditional Sail Order" in place.[202] The Conditional Sail Order would require industry to demonstrate through a series of incremental steps—including completing simulated voyages using mitigation best practices and building a sufficient testing program—that they could safely resume passenger operations before they were permitted to sail.[203] Dr. Cetron noted that Dr. Redfield returned from a White House Coronavirus Task Force meeting and informed him that a Conditional Sail Order is "where we landed" and directed him "to rewrite everything[.]"[204] Given the scope of these preliminary requirements, Dr. Redfield said that he did not believe at the time that any cruise line would be able to satisfy these requirements within "a year."[205]

Dr. Redfield acknowledged that "a lot of people" "were angry" about the agency's decision to implement a Conditional Sail Order, including "your Florida Senators, your Florida governor," who questioned why a conditional order was needed.[206] Dr. Redfield told the Select Subcommittee that he "felt very strongly" about the need to stand firm against these calls to let the No Sail Order expire altogether—particularly after he had allowed CDC's testing guidance to be compromised—and recognized that he could be fired for issuing the Conditional Sail Order:

> Even if the Task Force said I wasn't signing it, I was signing it. And if that meant that I was resigning or being fired as CDC Director, that was going to happen. . . . I already made the concession on asymptomatic spread, and had to reverse that, that I wasn't budging on this. And if it meant a Corona White House Task Force said we weren't going to extend it, as CDC director, I was going to sign it and extend it, and assumed this would be the last thing I did as CDC director.[207]

With the Conditional Sail Order in place, followed by the authorization of safe and effective coronavirus vaccines, commercial sailing resumed in 2021. Reflecting on this outcome, Dr. Cetron told the Select Subcommittee that the Conditional Sail Order ultimately was "a way to provide both what the government thought would be necessary to assure a safer pathway" than acquiescing to calls to abandon a No Sail Order altogether, as well as a vehicle for "providing some future clear direction to an industry."[208]

IV. Trump Administration Officials Repeatedly Sought to Influence and Block CDC Scientific Reports for Political Purposes

Trump Administration officials engaged in a wide-reaching campaign to manipulate the substance and block the dissemination of accurate scientific information related to the coronavirus—with the apparent goal of helping President Trump politically. From at least May to mid-September 2020, senior HHS officials attempted to alter or suppress at least 19 different CDC scientific reports that they deemed to be politically harmful to President Trump's perceived political interests. These reports were primarily published in CDC's flagship publication, the MMWR, but HHS officials also interfered with at least one HAN advisory providing urgent public health information to clinicians. HHS officials also took unprecedented steps to insert political appointees into the publication process and rebut CDC's scientific reports, including drafting op-eds and other public messaging designed to directly counteract CDC's findings. Although CDC was able to stave off much of the pressure, Trump

Administration political appointees were successful in their efforts to make changes and delay the release of multiple scientific reports.

A. HHS Officials Successfully Interfered with an MMWR to Downplay Evidence of Early Spread of the Coronavirus

The Select Subcommittee released evidence in December 2020 demonstrating that Mr. Caputo and Dr. Alexander pressured CDC to change the title of an MMWR regarding the spread of the coronavirus from Europe in the early months of 2020 in a manner that downplayed the report's key finding. Specifically, on May 21, 2020, Dr. Alexander wrote to Mr. Hall that he believed the MMWR was "misleading and little inflamming [sic]" and sought to change the title and insert language praising what he called the Trump Administration's "[s]trong mitigation and containment measures."[209] Although CDC did not add the reference to the Administration's actions to the MMWR, they changed the title to read: "Evidence of **Limited** Early Spread of COVID-19 Within the United States, January–February 2020."[210]

New documents reveal that Dr. Redfield personally coordinated with Mr. Caputo about altering the MMWR and related press materials in an apparent effort to make them more politically palatable. On May 23, 2020, Dr. Redfield sent Mr. Caputo an updated draft of the MMWR, highlighting the change to the title and asking if he had additional comments. Mr. Caputo forwarded the draft to Dr. Alexander, who indicated that he was pleased with the changes:[211]

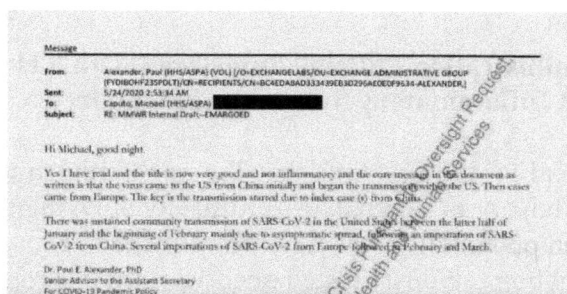

> Yes I have read and the title is now very good and not inflammatory and the core message in this document as written is that the virus came to the US from China initially and began the transmission with the US.

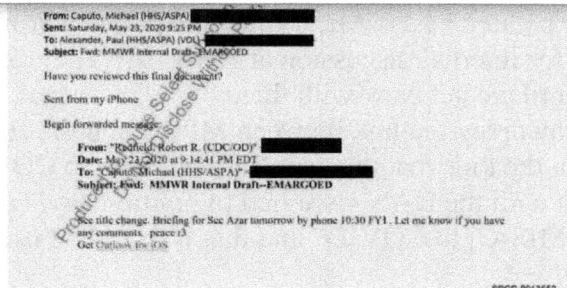

Dr. Alexander also wrote to Mr. Caputo the next day to raise concerns about the press materials:

> The issue I raise is that here you have the CDC officially stating that the cases from Europe were a likely cause or contributed to the spread in the US. The media and naysayers would ask why did the President not close Europe at the same time he closed China Jan 31…or why not soon after? Why wait till March?

Dr. Alexander proposed changes to three documents and indicated that he was worried the press materials, if left unchanged, would cause "the media [to] go after" the Administration. Mr. Caputo forwarded the email to Dr. Redfield and asked what he thought about Dr. Alexander's concerns, to which Dr. Redfield replied: "I agree with Paul." Mr. Caputo also agreed, calling the press materials "misleading and even provocative," concluding: "That language has to be improved."[212] The next day, Dr. Alexander sent the proposed changes to the press documents to a larger group of HHS and CDC officials.[213]

Previously undisclosed internal correspondence sheds light on the Trump Administration's sensitivity about the MMWR. At Dr. Redfield's request, Secretary Azar received a "careful brief" on the report prior to its release[214]—possibly due to a similar MMWR that had angered Trump Administration officials earlier in the month.[215] On May 24, 2020, Dr. Redfield circulated an updated draft of the MMWR to a group of senior public health officials, noting that "Changes have been made as discussed on our call this morning." The revised version of the MMWR was released on June 5.[216]

B. Trump Administration Officials Interfered with a Health Alert on Multisystem Inflammatory Syndrome in Children

New documents reveal for the first time that Trump Administration officials interfered in the publication of a HAN advisory in May 2020—ultimately delaying the release of a report that warned of MIS-C, a new and potentially fatal condition similar to Kawasaki disease that was identified in some children who previously tested positive for the coronavirus.[217] HAN advisories are used to disseminate pressing information to public health practitioners, clinicians, and laboratories.[218]

On May 13, 2020, CDC sent a draft of the HAN advisory seeking immediate clearance to facilitate its release on an expedited basis. Mr. Caputo instructed a group of HHS officials to "Hold this please" to allow for internal discussion at HHS. Mr. Hall replied confirming that he told CDC "to hold on this until we get back with them."[219] Dr. Alexander concurrently sent edits to the advisory seeking to downplay the link between MIS-C and the coronavirus, claiming that there was not "a clear link in the kids that the one death was due to COVID."[220] Dr. Alexander made clear that his concerns with the HAN were tied to politics, saying "the media and folk with agendas are trying to tie it [MIS-C] to COVID" and that it would be used to "blame the administration."[221]

The next day, Mr. Hall instructed CDC to "hold on all interviews on this for now."[222] CDC ultimately released the HAN advisory later that afternoon.[223] Afterwards, Dr. Alexander emailed Mr. Murphy asking whether changes could be made to the advisory after it had been released—attempting to revise the language to state that the patients initially tested negative for the coronavirus when admitted to the hospital.[224] HAN staff pushed back on the suggestion, telling Mr. Hall that the statement in the advisory was accurate.[225]

C. HHS Officials Attempted to Shelve and Rebut an MMWR Discrediting Hydroxychloroquine

As outlined in a December 21, 2020, letter, the Select Subcommittee uncovered extensive evidence of efforts by senior HHS officials to interfere with the publication of an MMWR detailing the significant growth of hydroxychloroquine prescriptions during the pandemic.[226] The MMWR found that the number of prescriptions for hydroxychloroquine increased 80-fold between March 2019 and March 2020, despite a lack of data showing the efficacy of the drug for treating the coronavirus and evidence that it increased the risk of serious adverse events.[227]

During a transcribed interview, Ms. Witkofsky recounted that Mr. Caputo expressed concern over the MMWR because he "knew it was going to cause a lot of media" attention and asked her to check when it would be released.[228] In response, Ms. Witkofsky obtained the full-length, pre-print draft of the MMWR and provided it to Dr. Alexander and Mr. Caputo—violating longstanding CDC practice to not circulate pre-production drafts outside of the agency.[229] Dr. Walke explained that this practice serves to "protect the integrity of the document, or scientific integrity of the publication and MMWR" and "to provide a buffer from any political interference in the editorial process."[230]

Dr. Alexander and Mr. Caputo—who championed the use of hydroxychloroquine as a coronavirus treatment even after the Food and Drug Administration (FDA) revoked its emergency use authorization[231]—sought to edit and prevent publication of this report. After receiving a copy of the MMWR draft, Dr. Alexander sent an email to Mr. Caputo and Ms. Witkofsky, saying "Hi Michael, is this not the article we were shelving?"[232] The following day, Mr. Caputo's assistant, Madeleine Hubbard, told Ms. Witkofsky that they had "quite a few edits" and asked to be kept "in the loop on this MMWR."[233]

On July 2, 2020, Ms. Hubbard sent a draft op-ed attacking the report to Mr. Caputo and Mr. Alexander. That document—which does not appear to have been published—argued that the MMWR "presents factual information with an agenda" and could "prevent the news from giving the proper coverage of a true 'miracle cure.'" The rebuttal also asserted that "there is no academic value in this study whatsoever" and slandered the authors of the MMWR, calling them "a disgrace to public service" and accusing them of being "self-aggrandizing, looking to grab headlines" and "ignoring and [sic] the Americans currently dying from COVID-19."[234]

Dr. Charlotte Kent, the Editor-in-Chief of the MMWR, told the Select Subcommittee during a transcribed interview that she was not aware of the rebuttal at the time, but that the release of such a document by HHS was "not typical" and "could undermine confidence in CDC and in the quality of science that is in MMWR."[235] The MMWR, originally scheduled for release on June 30, 2020, was not published until September 4.[236]

D. HHS Officials Attempted to Edit, Rebut, and Delay the Release of an MMWR Regarding an Outbreak at a Georgia Summer Camp

The Select Subcommittee previously released extensive evidence of a coordinated effort by Trump Administration appointees to blunt the potential political impact of an MMWR regarding a coronavirus outbreak at a Georgia summer camp.[237] On July 27, 2020, Dr. Alexander sent Dr. Kent an email criticizing a summary of the MMWR, stating:[238]

> This CDC MMWR also concluded by saying in spite of adhering to CDC guidance, the spread was massive, with elevated attack rates. . . . the piece reads as if CDC's own guidance is not adequate and that even if a school or similar implements most recommended strategies to prevent transmission, that there will still be massive spread. . . . It just sends the wrong message as written and actually reads as if to send a message of NOT to re-open

CDC officials agreed to revise the MMWR in response to Dr. Alexander's comments, as well as additional comments from Dr. Redfield.[239] In an email, Dr. Kent told Dr. Alexander:

> In response to thoughtful comments from CDC leadership and you, the opening sentence of Georgia's report has been reframed. The opening sentence was the only reference to schools or institutions of higher learning in the report, and reference to them has been removed.[240]

A new document obtained by the Select Subcommittee reveals that on July 28, 2020, Ms. Witkofsky breached the CDC protocol against circulating draft MMWRs outside the agency by providing a complete draft of the MMWR directly to Dr. Alexander and other HHS officials. Following Ms. Witkofsky's acknowledgment that CDC planned to release a proactive statement to accompany the public release of the MMWR, Dr. Alexander made clear that his concerns about the MMWR were political in nature, saying, "Based on that report I cant [sic] see anything positive being said." He also leveled the accusation that "This is meant to send a message or put out a message that is not right."[241]

HHS officials coordinated to rebut the report's key finding that children can transmit the virus to each other and to adults. At Mr. Caputo's direction, Dr. Alexander drafted an op-ed seeking to downplay the risk of children transmitting the coronavirus and that sought to provide "very re-assuring information and even for the White House."[242] The op-ed went through several drafts at HHS, with Mr. Caputo and other senior HHS officials providing comments.[243] Although the draft op-ed went into the clearance process at HHS,[244] it does not appear to have been published. Dr. Alexander repeatedly urged its publication during the early weeks of August 2020, asserting that "[t]he piece is less about numbers but to tell a good story" and that the goal behind the piece was "to give good news."[245] During a transcribed interview, Mr. Hall stated that HHS's efforts to rebut the MMWR were "out of the ordinary" and that he could not recall another instance during his 23 years at HHS in which someone from ASPA had written an opinion piece rebutting something put out by CDC.[246]

The initial release of the Georgia summer camp MMWR, originally set for July 29, 2020, was delayed to July 31 at the direction of Dr. Redfield and HHS.[247] According to Dr. Kent, the delay was due to Dr. Redfield's scheduled testimony before the Select Subcommittee on the morning of July 31.[248] Dr. Redfield did not discuss the MMWR's findings at the July 31 hearing,[249] and the MMWR was released approximately fifteen minutes after its conclusion.[250] CDC officials told the Select Subcommittee that delaying an MMWR until after a congressional hearing was unusual. According to Rear Admiral Michael Iademarco, Director of CDC's Center for Surveillance, Epidemiology, and Laboratory Services who supervises the MMWR Editor-in-Chief, it is "not common" for MMWRs to be delayed close to their intended publication date.[251] When asked for his recollection about the delayed publication of this MMWR, Dr. Redfield said, "I really don't remember what that was about," adding, "I wouldn't think that it had anything to do with me testifying, since I -- you know, I'm very comfortable telling people the truth when I'm asked to testify."[252]

E. Trump Officials Instructed CDC Employees to Destroy Evidence of Political Interference

In a December 10, 2020, letter, the Select Subcommittee released evidence of Dr. Alexander's significant escalation of his efforts to interfere with CDC's publication of MMWRs on August 8, 2020—in which he demanded that HHS receive unprecedented power to make changes to reports prior to publication in an attempt to benefit the perceived political interests of the former president. In a new email obtained by the Select Subcommittee sent earlier that same day, Dr. Alexander wrote to Mr. Caputo, Ms. Witkofsky, and a number of HHS political appointees railing against an MMWR on coronavirus risks to children. Dr. Alexander outlined concerns that he had with the MMWR and accused CDC of "corruptness in the reporting," stating:[253]

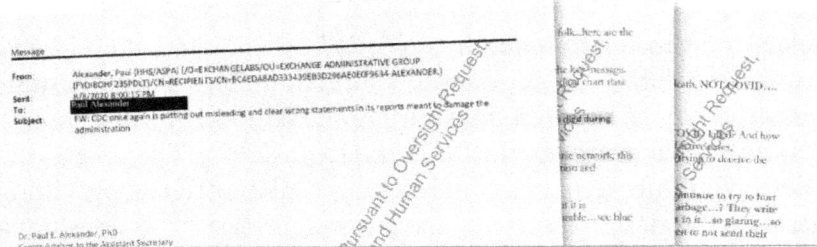

It is so false how they reported this and other reports…I don't understand why they continue to try to hurt the public and the administration…the summary is so misleading. Who writes this garbage…?
. . . This is about scaring parents and women to hide in the basement and to impact the election…again, to damage the administration. . . . CDC needs to be schooled and cleaned up. It is rogue or seems so or If I were to see an agency doing the things CDC is doing and how they are reporting etc., I would conclude they are rouge [sic] and up to mischief in their reporting.

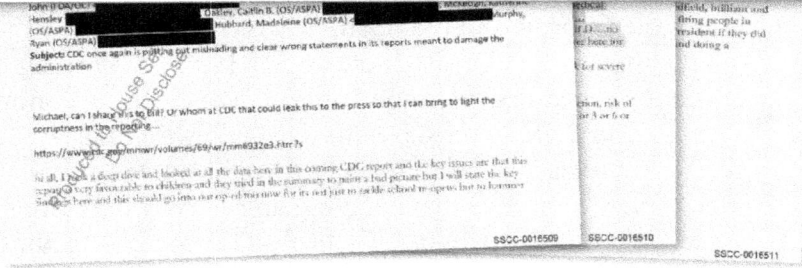

In a subsequent email to Dr. Redfield, Mr. Caputo, Dr. Kent, and other officials at CDC and ASPA released in November 2021, Dr. Alexander repeated similar accusations against CDC, including claiming that CDC officials were writing MMWRs that were "hit pieces on the administration," "very misleading," and "designed to hurt this Presidnet [sic]." Dr. Alexander insisted that CDC alter or rescind the MMWR on coronavirus risks to children and the Georgia summer camp report, which he suggested were damaging to President Trump. He also demanded that CDC change its process for releasing MMWRs, so that he would have the opportunity to review and make changes to draft reports in advance of publication, or otherwise HHS should stop the publication of all future MMWRs:

> I am asking that you put an **immediate stop** on all CDC MMWR reports due to the incompleteness of reporting that is done in a manner to mislead the public . . . . Nothing to go out unless I read and agree with the findings how they CDC, wrote it and I tweak it to ensure it is fair and balanced and "complete". And not misleading.[254]

Numerous CDC officials told the Select Subcommittee that they were troubled by Dr. Alexander's demand to shut down production of the MMWR. Dr. Christine Casey, Editor of the MMWR Serials, stated that she found it "highly unusual and quite concerning for somebody to ask to put an immediate stop on MMWR reports. I don't think in my memory that has ever happened."[255] Dr. Walke believed "[t]his was -- this would be a red line, I think, for all of us."[256] Dr. Iademarco similarly explained that he thought the email "crosses a line."[257]

During a transcribed interview, Dr. Casey recounted that she was so alarmed when she received Dr. Alexander's August 8, 2020, email that she called and woke up Dr. Iademarco—who supervised her own boss—at approximately 2 a.m. After discussing the email, Dr. Casey and Dr. Iademarco decided to reach out to Dr. Redfield. Dr. Casey emailed Dr. Redfield and other senior CDC officials in the early morning hours of August 9, stating that she and Dr. Iademarco were "available to discuss next steps with you and OD [Office of the Director] leadership (copied) in the morning."[258]

Dr. Casey told the Select Subcommittee that she connected with Dr. Iademarco mid-morning on August 9, 2020. According to Dr. Casey:

> [Dr. Iademarco] informed me that he had communicated with the director [Dr. Redfield], and that I was to—that the action of doing nothing was what we were going to do. And he asked me to delete the email, instructed me to delete the email.

When asked what Dr. Iademarco had specifically said, Dr. Casey responded: "I believe he said that the director said to delete the email, and that anyone else who had received it, you know, should do as well."[259]

Dr. Casey described the instruction to delete the email as "unusual" and that it "made [her] uncomfortable" because she had never been instructed to delete an email before.[260] Dr. Casey stated that she ultimately "followed the instruction in my chain of command" and deleted the email from her inbox. She confirmed that she also relayed the instruction to delete the email to Dr. Kent and another CDC official.[261] Before deleting the email, Dr. Casey printed a hard copy in order to "satisfy [her] personal discomfort," and as a way of "retaining and preserving the record."[262] Dr. Kent affirmed that Dr. Casey instructed her to delete Dr. Alexander's email and that she understood the deletion request had come from Dr. Redfield.[263]

When asked about this incident, Dr. Iademarco said that he did not recall Dr. Redfield using the word "delete" in connection with this email and did not recall telling Dr. Casey to delete the email from Dr. Alexander.[264] Dr. Redfield told the Select Subcommittee that he never gave an instruction to delete Dr. Alexander's email, instead he "made it clear at the CDC that they should just ignore [Dr.] Alexander's emails."[265]

F. Trump Administration Officials Succeeded in Their Attempts to Interfere with CDC's Scientific Publications

The Select Subcommittee's investigation has revealed that senior HHS officials attempted to alter the contents, rebut, or delay the release of at least 19 scientific reports from CDC related to the pandemic:

- A May 14, 2020, HAN advisory regarding MIS-C, which was delayed for a day at Mr. Caputo's instruction (detailed above);[266]

- A May 29 MMWR regarding early spread of the coronavirus (detailed above);[267]

- A June 5 MMWR regarding coronavirus prevention practices;[268]

- A June 12 MMWR regarding public attitudes related to stay-at-home orders, nonessential business closures, and public health guidance;[269]

- A June 12 MMWR regarding national case surveillance and demographic characteristics, reported symptoms, underlying health conditions, and outcomes among patients with the coronavirus;[270]

- A June 26 MMWR regarding characteristics of women of reproductive age with coronavirus infection and risks to pregnant women;[271]

- A June 30 MMWR regarding characteristics of adult inpatients and outpatients with coronavirus infection;[272]

- An MMWR regarding hydroxychloroquine prescription trends, originally scheduled for release on June 30 but not published until September 4 (detailed above);[273]

- A July 14 MMWR on the use of cloth face coverings among adults during the pandemic;[274]

- A July 24 MMWR regarding underlying medical conditions associated with the risk of severe COVID-19;[275]

- A July 31 MMWR, originally scheduled for release on July 29, regarding a coronavirus outbreak at a Georgia summer camp (detailed above);[276]

- A July 31 MMWR regarding efforts to mitigate coronavirus transmission during the April 7 primary election in Milwaukee, Wisconsin;[277]

- A July 31 MMWR regarding vaccination among children in New York City during the pandemic;[278]

- An August 14 MMWR, originally scheduled for release on August 7, regarding hospitalization rates for children diagnosed with the coronavirus (detailed above);[279]

- An August 14 MMWR, originally scheduled for release on August 7, regarding MIS-C;[280]

- A September 4 MMWR regarding coronavirus outbreaks at four summer camps in Maine;[281]

- A September 18 MMWR on coronavirus-associated deaths among children, adolescents, and young adults;[282]

- An October 5 MMWR regarding a coronavirus outbreak caused by a 13-year-old, the title of which was altered following a suggestion from Dr. Giroir;[283] and

- A December 2 MMWR adopting recommendations from the Advisory Committee on Immunization Practices regarding the allocation of initial supplies of the coronavirus vaccine which Secretary Azar requested—via two separate phone calls to Dr. Redfield—be rejected.[284]

Although CDC officials told the Select Subcommittee that the agency was able to withstand Trump Administration officials' attempts to influence CDC's scientific reports and that the scientific integrity of the MMWR was ultimately not impacted,[285] the Select Subcommittee found that HHS political appointees succeeded in altering or delaying the release of at least five scientific reports. As revealed in an April 9, 2021, letter sent by the Select Subcommittee, Dr. Alexander boasted in an August 30, 2020, email to Ms. Witkofsky, that there had been an apparent shift in the tenor of MMWR articles after she became CDC Acting Chief of Staff earlier that month:[286]

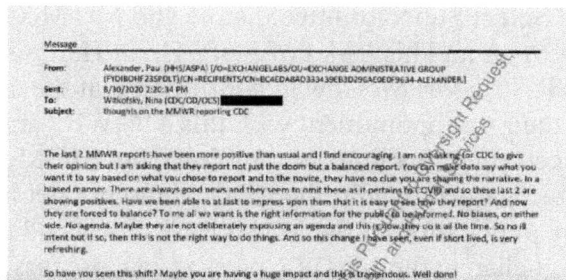

> The last 2 MMWR reports have been more positive than usual and I find encouraging . . . . Have we been able to at last to [sic] impress upon them that it is easy to see how they report? And now they are forced to balance? …. So have you seen this shift? Maybe you are having a huge impact and this is tremendous. Well done!

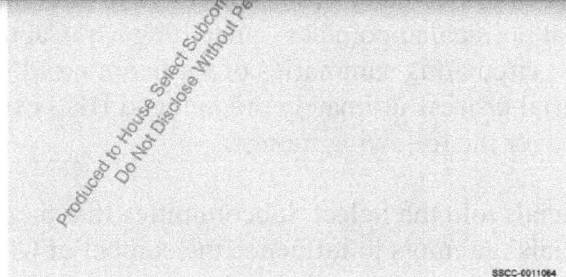

On September 9, Dr. Alexander bragged to Mr. Caputo about two "[e]xamples of CDC adjusting writing based on my inquiry," calling it a "small victory but a victory nonetheless and yippee!!!"[287]

Trump Administration appointees also succeeded in pressuring CDC to change the editorial process of the MMWR. Prior to the pandemic, officials outside of CDC played no role in the editorial or publication process of the MMWR—with pre-production drafts and abstracts or summaries of MMWRs not circulated outside of the agency and HHS officials having no ability to seek to make changes to MMWRs.[288] During a transcribed interview, Dr. Schuchat explained it was a "longstanding practice that the MMWRs are scientific products of CDC, and that there's a firewall between the editorial production and political levels."[289]

This changed during the pandemic after Trump Administration officials were reportedly upset that an MMWR written by Dr. Schuchat detailing the steps that HHS had taken in January and February 2020 to address the coronavirus "did not draw the conclusion sought by the Administration—i.e., that everything that could have been done was done."[290] Dr. Schuchat told the Select Subcommittee that she received "negative feedback" from within the Administration and was made aware of "conversations at HHS and at the White House about concerns about the MMWR." In particular, Dr. Schuchat received a phone call from White House Chief of Staff Mark Meadows regarding the MMWR which left her feeling "very shaken."[291] She said that this was the only time in her 33-year career at CDC that a White House Chief of Staff had ever contacted her to discuss a CDC report.[292]

Dr. Redfield told the Select Subcommittee that he and Mr. McGowan also received a weekend call from Secretary Azar and his Chief of Staff, Brian Harrison, both of whom were "not happy about the MMWR."[293] Mr. McGowan confirmed that the call occurred, saying the officials sought to "express their disappointment with this MMWR" and that Secretary Azar specifically was "upset." According to a joint submission from Mr. McGowan and Ms. Campbell, Secretary Azar warned that "if the CDC would not get in line, then HHS would take control of approving the publication of the MMWRs." They said that after Dr. Redfield indicated that CDC would not change the MMWR peer review process, Secretary Azar and HHS General Counsel Robert Charrow "directed CDC to change the MMWR process and added that if CDC did not follow the directive, then HHS would take MMWRs away from the CDC or stop their publication."[294]

CDC ultimately acceded to Secretary Azar's directive to alter the MMWR process. Ms. Campbell added external political appointees—including Mr. Caputo and Dr. Alexander—to CDC's email distribution list circulating summaries of forthcoming MMWRs in May 2020.[295] This change to CDC's editorial process ultimately precipitated HHS officials' attempts to interfere with the MMWRs over the following months.

Numerous CDC officials told the Select Subcommittee that they were deeply troubled by Trump Administration officials' attempts to influence the content of CDC's scientific reports and to subvert the historically independent process for disseminating public health information through MMWRs. For instance:

- Dr. Schuchat told the Select Subcommittee that the efforts by Dr. Alexander and HHS officials to influence MMWRs caused her "many concerns," because "it didn't seem appropriate for political appointees in communication to be involved in that effort."[296]

- Dr. Casey said that Dr. Alexander's efforts were "unprecedented" and "breached" the "production firewall" put in place to protect the independence and integrity of the MMWR.[297]

- Dr. Walke called Dr. Alexander's attempts to influence the MMWR process "ridiculous, and such an overreach," remarking "how dare he." Dr. Walke added that he was worried Dr. Alexander's interference "would be the end of the MMWR, and all of our scientific integrity if he was allowed to review and edit CDC publications." [298]

- According to a veteran of the Commissioned Corps of the U.S. Public Health Service and Epidemic Intelligence Service, Dr. Kent admitted during a Zoom meeting in September 2020 that she threatened to resign publicly if the political interference continued at MMWR.[299]

Dr. Redfield also told the Select Subcommittee that he found Dr. Alexander's emails to be "inappropriate" and told Mr. Caputo that the emails should "stop." Dr. Redfield said that he told Mr. Caputo on multiple occasions that "he [Dr. Alexander] was not helpful to the CDC, and I didn't want him bothering the CDC people anymore," and that "he [Mr. Caputo] needed to get rid of him."[300]

It does not appear that any action was taken to stop the pervasive attempts by Trump Administration political appointees to interfere with CDC's publication of scientific reports until after CDC received press inquiries on Dr. Alexander's interference with MMWRs in September 2020.[301] In December 2020, the Select Subcommittee released an email showing that on September 9, a reporter from *Politico* reached out to HHS seeking comment on concerns regarding Dr. Alexander.[302] Two days later, on September 11, Ms. Witkofsky instructed Dr. Kent to remove Dr. Alexander—but not Mr. Caputo—from the MMWR summary email distribution list.[303] During a transcribed interview, Ms. Witkofsky explained that she gave this instruction "because of all the comments and crazy stuff he [Dr. Alexander] wrote."[304]

New emails reveal that, despite these admonitions, Dr. Alexander continued pushing Mr. Caputo to make changes to MMWRs and for HHS to take a larger role in overseeing the MMWR publication process.[305] In a September 13, 2020, email, Dr. Alexander wrote: "I am making a formal request for CDC to provide us with complete reports when asking for our clearance and input. . . . We must also be allowed ample time to review before publishing." He also called for HHS to "officially conduct a review of all CDC MMWR reporting in the last 6 months for this COVID pandemic" because he claimed that "the conclusions or message by CDC at times do not match the underlying data."[306] Although Mr. Caputo had previously expressed approval over Dr. Alexander's attempts to influence CDC's publications, Mr. Caputo responded to a separate email that Dr. Alexander sent, saying:[307]

Are you watching the news today? Your email demands of the CDC are leading every network news program and will lead the Sunday shows. Every major newspaper too. This is not a good place for you to be - and you put me there too. Do you think this is a job well done? Don't send any emails to anyone outside ASPA until further notice.

HHS announced on September 16, 2020, that Dr. Alexander had left his position at HHS and that Mr. Caputo would take a medical leave of absence.[308] Dr. Alexander continued to send emails to CDC staff seeking to make changes to MMWRs even after his departure.[309]

V. The Trump Administration Wasted Millions of Taxpayer Dollars on a Failed Celebrity Vanity Campaign

Soon after being appointed to lead HHS's public affairs office amid a worsening pandemic, Mr. Caputo began conversations with the Trump White House about organizing a large-scale taxpayer-funded coronavirus public advertising campaign.[310] These discussions culminated in a $265 million federal campaign that internal HHS contracting documents show sought to harness "the power of traditional, digital and social media" to "[d]efeat despair and inspire hope."[311]

The campaign contemplated two phases: A six-month "immediate surge" phase for which a nearly $15 million contract was awarded to consulting firm Atlas Research (Atlas), and a "short term" phase for which a $251 million contract was awarded to Fors Marsh Group.[312] The immediate surge phase of the campaign was centered on a series of public service announcements (PSAs) featuring celebrities and other high-profile influencers discussing the federal response to the coronavirus alongside federal public health officials.[313] The campaign schedule contemplated releasing an ad blitz in the weeks leading up to the November 2020 presidential election.

Trump Administration officials used hundreds of millions of dollars from CDC's budget to pay for what amounted to a celebrity vanity campaign—which one former HHS official reportedly said raised "every red flag I could dream of."[314] In the process, millions of taxpayer dollars were earmarked for handpicked private-sector allies of Mr. Caputo. Members of the campaign team proceeded to vet celebrities based on whether they supported President Trump or Democratic politicians and political causes, while Mr. Caputo sought to inject overtly pro-Trump slogans—such as "Helping the President Will Help the Country"—into the campaign messaging.

A. Mr. Caputo Was a Driving Force Behind the Immediate Surge Campaign, Which Raided CDC's Budget and Intended to Spend the "Vast Majority" of Its Funds Before the Presidential Election

Within weeks of arriving at HHS, Mr. Caputo set out to build a large-scale public messaging campaign to "defeat despair and inspire hope" in Americans heading into the fall of 2020.[315] In a transcribed interview with the Select Subcommittee, HHS Deputy Assistant for Public Affairs Mark Weber—a 32-year career HHS official—said that Mr. Caputo was engaging in discussions with White House officials about a coronavirus public relations campaign as early as June 2020. According to Mr. Weber, Mr. Caputo and Michael Pratt—a senior HHS political appointee—developed and presented to the White House a one-page document that outlined the goals of this campaign.[316] Mr. Weber said that he was soon tasked by Mr. Caputo with executing a campaign consistent with these goals.[317] Mr. Weber told the Select Subcommittee that Mr. Caputo oversaw the campaign and implemented "his vision of how this campaign was going to operate."[318]

The White House tapped into CDC's budget to fund the ASPA-led initiative. Mr. Weber said that Mr. Caputo informed him on or around July 9, 2020, that ASPA would receive approximately $300 million for the campaign pursuant to an interagency agreement with CDC.[319] Congress had appropriated these funds to CDC for coronavirus relief purposes, but they were rerouted to ASPA instead.[320] Dr. Redfield told the Select Subcommittee that he was not provided a reason why CDC's funds were reprogrammed for ASPA's campaign and noted that he "wasn't a happy camper reprogramming money from CDC for another initiative."[321] Although CDC's budget was used to fund the effort and the agency historically supported a variety of major public health education campaigns, no CDC officials were included on or involved in the campaign team, according to Mr. Weber and Dr. Redfield—despite the fact that officials from other key HHS subagencies, such as FDA and the National Institutes of Health, were added.[322]

Mr. Weber said he was approached by John "Wolf" Wagner—a political appointee at FDA and close ally of Mr. Caputo[323]—in late July 2020 about using an FDA contract as a vehicle for funding the immediate surge phase of the campaign.[324] An FDA contract was ultimately identified and used, but Mr. Weber said that ASPA oversaw and managed the campaign at all times.[325] On August 5, FDA issued a final solicitation for this phase titled "COVID-19 Immediate Surge Public Service Advertising and Awareness Campaign," which stipulated that the "vast majority" of the contract's $15 million budget was expected to be spent "in the first two months" of the project—which was scheduled for August and September, in the direct lead up to the November presidential election.[326]

B. Mr. Caputo's Outside Allies Were Classified as "Preferred Subcontractors"

Weeks before the federal government issued an award for the immediate surge contract, Mr. Caputo took steps to bring close personal allies into the campaign team.[327] In a July 19, 2020, email newly released by the Select Subcommittee, Mr. Caputo contacted a group of individuals inside and outside of government regarding a "public health communications initiative."[328] One such individual was Den Tolmor, Mr. Caputo's longtime friend and business partner.[329] Mr. Tolmor was reportedly one of Mr. Caputo's private-sector clients as recently as April 2020 and had paid Mr. Caputo at least $5,000 to handle his public relations.[330] Mr. Caputo was also reported to be the chief marketing officer of an online video streaming platform that Mr. Tolmor founded.[331] In the July 19 email, Mr. Caputo wrote: "I'm really looking forward to getting our public health communications initiative moving in the days ahead" and called for the group to "embark on this historic journey together."[332] In response, a representative of the advertising company Grapeseed Media noted that they had already begun work to "develop the targeting, story, and creative messaging for the public communications campaign"—even though the contract would not be awarded for more than a month.[333]

Mr. Weber told the Select Subcommittee that he became aware of Mr. Caputo's prior relationship with Mr. Tolmor during conversations with another contractor regarding Mr. Tolmor's company, DD&T Group LLC (DD&T).[334] Upon learning of this connection, Mr. Weber said that he approached Mr. Caputo to discuss the issue.[335] Mr. Weber explained that he was concerned at the time about "the appearance of improper business relationships or improper procurements" and wanted Mr. Caputo "to be very aware that this relationship could turn into something—a distraction from the important work that needed to be done."[336] Mr. Weber said that Mr. Caputo responded to these concerns by saying, "let's proceed" with using DD&T for the campaign.[337]

Following Mr. Caputo's instruction, HHS decided to list Mr. Caputo's favored firms, including DD&T and Grapeseed Media, as the federal government's "preferred subcontractors" in the FDA solicitation for proposals.[338] According to Mr. Weber, "there really was no choice" other than to list the preferred subcontractors in the FDA solicitation. Mr. Weber elaborated that HHS listed these favored firms in the solicitation for proposals because "you just cannot hire individuals that you want to work with. There has got to be an open, competitive process that is documented," and HHS believed that this arrangement satisfied those obligations.[339]

On August 4, 2020, FDA issued a draft solicitation for the immediate surge contract to Atlas, listing three "preferred subcontractors" in the solicitation whom FDA described as "uniquely positioned" for the campaign: DD&T, Grapeseed Media, and Co/efficient, a market research company run by a Republican pollster.[340] According to the findings of a GAO investigation into the contract, ASPA wanted to execute a sole source contract with Atlas— rather than allowing other firms to compete for the award—but agreed to solicit a proposal from one other firm after FDA recommended they do so. GAO's investigation found that Atlas agreed to hire Mr. Caputo's three preferred subcontractors in its proposal, but the other firm solicited did not.[341] HHS ultimately awarded the immediate surge contract to Atlas over the other firm in late August 2020.[342] An email previously released by the Select Subcommittee, the Committee on Oversight and Reform, and the Subcommittee on Economic and Consumer Policy as part of a joint investigation[343] shows that Atlas representatives acknowledged to ASPA that they hired the preferred subcontractors at the "encouragement" of the Trump Administration.[344] A copy of the DD&T subcontract obtained in the joint investigation and newly released reveals that Mr. Tolmor's company stood to make more than $1.4 million over a period of six months for its work on the campaign.[345]

An internal company document released in October 2020 shows that Atlas employees expressed concerns about the qualifications of Mr. Caputo's preferred subcontractors. On August 14, 2020, Atlas's President sent an email documenting diligence the firm ran on the subcontractors, which found that all three were "[s]mall shops with little on them in the public domain." In particular, the diligence found "nothing at all on DD&T Group as a corporate entity," other than it was "an LLC platform owned by Den Tolmor, a Russia-born business associate of Caputo's." Given the subcontractors' limited track records, Atlas's President wrote that the company needed to have a "backup plan in place in the event one of the three subs cannot perform."[346]

In his transcribed interview, Mr. Weber could not recall any other specific instance in his 32-year career at HHS where another solicitation enumerated "preferred subcontractors."[347] FDA officials similarly told GAO investigators that "it was unusual for firms to be suggested as potential subcontractors during the solicitation phase."[348] After conducting a review of the immediate surge contract, GAO took the extraordinary step earlier this year of making a referral to the HHS Office of Inspector General and DOJ in light of "a potential pre-existing business relationship between an ASPA official involved in the public education campaign and one of the suggested subcontractors."[349]

C. The White House Closely Monitored the Timing of the Campaign, as Mr. Caputo Pressed to Move Faster

According to Mr. Weber, White House National Economic Council Director Larry Kudlow was "constantly interested in progress" on the campaign after it began. Mr. Weber told the Select Subcommittee that Mr. Kudlow regularly called Mr. Caputo "to see where we were with the campaign"—initially calling as often as every week.[350] Mr. Kudlow's primary concern was the timing of the campaign, including when the White House would start to see ads running.[351]

Mr. Caputo pressed the campaign team to quickly film PSAs with celebrity influencers, insisting in a September 2020 email to the campaign team that "we must film them ASAP—we need content in the can now."[352] Throughout this period, Mr. Caputo sought to exercise unilateral decision making for key aspects of the campaign and directed his preferred subcontractors to engage in specific tasks without the contracting officer's knowledge. For example, evidence obtained during the joint investigation shows that Mr. Caputo:

- Held individual meetings with Mr. Tolmor to discuss the content of the campaign, including compiling lists of celebrities for the campaign team to vet and pursue, according to newly released documents.[353]

- Advised Mr. Tolmor to interface directly with Mr. Caputo's assistant, Ms. Hubbard, regarding the campaign, rather than going through the prime contractor or contracting officer, according to newly released text messages.[354]

- Contacted Grapeseed Media and attempted to insert himself into "the review process" as they were drafting a digital strategy for a component of the campaign, based on emails previously released by the Select Subcommittee.[355]

- Unilaterally instructed contractors as to which celebrities were "approved" for inclusion in the campaign, according to previously released documents.[356]

Mr. Weber said that he told Mr. Caputo that the contracting officer was "the only person who can assign work, approve work, and direct work of the contractors."[357] A previously released September 14, 2020, email from the HHS contracting officer to representatives of Atlas acknowledged that Atlas was "navigating a complex environment" in light of Mr. Caputo's conduct.[358]

D. Mr. Caputo Was Involved in Deploying Overtly Partisan Vetting Criteria and Sought to Inject Political Messaging into the Campaign

Evidence suggests that Mr. Caputo was also involved in developing and deploying overtly partisan vetting criteria to assess potential celebrities to participate in the campaign. A spreadsheet titled "PSA Celebrity Tracker" previously released during the joint investigation identified 274 celebrities and tracked their political affiliations and policy views. According to Mr. Weber, Mr. Tolmor was "an architect of the list" of potential celebrities. Mr. Weber said he assumed that Mr. Tolmor constructed this vetting document "working with Michael Caputo."[359]

The PSA Celebrity Tracker captured whether celebrities supported or had been critical of President Trump and whether they had supported Democratic political candidates or progressive policy issues, among other factors monitored. For example, the PSA Celebrity Tracker noted that George Lopez had made a "Controversial statement on President Trump in 2020"; Sean Penn "Publicly supports Democratic Party and candidates" and "Publicly supported same-sex marriage"; Christiana Aguilera is "an Obama-supporting Democrat and a gay-rights supporting liberal"; and Stephen Baldwin and Conor McGregor were each described as a "Public supporter of President Trump."[360]

Mr. Weber told the Select Subcommittee that the vetting criteria reflected in the PSA Celebrity Tracker was "very inconsistent" with the formal vetting guidance that was provided to Atlas.[361] According to Mr. Weber, vetting celebrities based on their support for the president in this manner would be "absolutely" inappropriate.[362] Contemporaneous notes prepared by Atlas and previously released indicate that the campaign team did not move forward with comedian George Lopez "due to previous concerns regarding his comments regarding the President"— seemingly a reference to the "Controversial statement on President Trump in 2020" that the vetting team flagged in the PSA Celebrity Tracker.[363] A separate celebrity tracking document obtained during the joint investigation also noted that both George Lopez and Sean Penn were "Not Recommended" for the campaign, the latter of whom was identified in the PSA Celebrity

Tracker as a supporter of the "Democratic Party and candidates."[364] A version of the PSA Celebrity Tracker—which included this overtly partisan vetting criteria—was emailed to certain ASPA officials working on the campaign in September 2020.[365]

Mr. Caputo also sought to push messaging for the campaign that contained overtly political components. Mr. Weber told the Select Subcommittee that Mr. Caputo presented "his vision for what the campaign could be" at a September 2020 meeting with contractors regarding the "messaging framework."[366] Contemporaneous notes from this meeting that were previously released captured multiple "Soundbites/Taglines" that made direct appeals to supporting President Trump:

- **"Helping the President will Help the Country**," which was described in the notes as a message that would "appeal to his base...."

- **"Keep America Well**," an apparent play on President Trump's 2020 campaign slogan, "Keep America Great."[367]

In his transcribed interview, Mr. Weber told the Select Subcommittee that these so-called taglines were "consistent with things that I heard Michael Caputo say." Mr. Weber stated that he felt that the slogans were "inconsistent with public health messaging" and not "consistent with science or public health."[368] During a September 13, 2020, Facebook Live video reported in the media, Mr. Caputo specifically tied the public relations campaign to President Trump's reelection prospects, asserting that the campaign was "demanded of me by the President of the United States. Personally," and stating that Democrats were "dead set against it" because "[t]hey cannot afford for us to have any good news before November because they're already losing."[369]

E. Millions of Taxpayer Dollars Were Wasted on the Failed Campaign

Mr. Caputo's celebrity PSA campaign was abandoned less than two months after the Trump Administration finalized the immediate surge contract, costing taxpayers millions of dollars. According to Mr. Weber, few celebrities were interested in working on the campaign, particularly amid growing concerns that the initiative was intended to benefit President Trump's reelection prospects.[370] An October 2020 progress report from Atlas that was previously released reflected that celebrities CeCe Winans and Dennis Quaid had "retracted consent to participate" in the campaign, and that the "[c]elebrities identified and approved as of 9/26 declined to participate due to negative press."[371] New text messages obtained in the joint investigation indicate that Mr. Tolmor had wanted the federal government to pay celebrities to participate in the campaign.[372]

Ultimately, only "two and a half" PSAs were filmed under the immediate surge contract.[373] After the Select Subcommittee launched a joint investigation into this matter along with the Committee on Oversight and Reform and Subcommittee on Economic and Consumer Policy, Secretary Azar announced that he ordered a "strategic review" of the campaign in October 2020.[374] The immediate surge contract was canceled the next month, after the review was completed.[375] Although no PSAs ever aired, GAO calculated that the federal government spent approximately $2.5 million under the immediate surge contract.[376]

VI. The Enduring Harms of the Trump Administration's Assault on the Nation's Public Health Institutions

The politicization of CDC by the Trump Administration took a significant toll on the agency's staff—including the career scientists working tirelessly to protect the nation during an unprecedented pandemic. By the fall of 2020, the Trump Administration's grip on CDC was so severe that one career official told the Select Subcommittee during a transcribed interview that it caused him to fear for his safety. Following a video rant by Mr. Caputo in September—during which he criticized the integrity of CDC scientists, accused CDC officials of plotting acts of sedition against President Trump, and encouraged supporters to stock up on ammunition[377]— Dr. Butler said, "one of the first things I did was look out my window at where the driveway was and how—where a truck bomb would be placed."[378]

Despite concerns over his own safety, Dr. Butler said that his "biggest concern was that there was intentional discrediting of the agency" which was "concerning given the level of the government that it was coming from." He described how the intentional discrediting of CDC adversely impacted morale at the agency:

> Working at CDC has always been something that many people have put a lot of pride in. . . . [P]eople who work there are so very committed to the people of America and really to global health. . . . But when people have committed to public service, it's really demoralizing to be characterized as a villain in the public health response, or even in the future of our country.[379]

The degree of control and hostility that the Trump Administration exerted over the historically independent agency not only demoralized CDC officials but also undermined Americans' trust in public health. In his transcribed interview, Dr. Cetron explained how this "erosion of credibility and trust really harms the ability to persuade people to take sometimes difficult steps that's in our joint collective interest"—steps that can be essential to preventing widespread loss of life when a society confronts a novel infectious disease like the coronavirus.[380] When asked if she believed that allowing CDC to convey accurate scientific advice to the public would have resulted in fewer Americans getting infected and dying during the early months of the pandemic, Dr. Schuchat told the Select Subcommittee:

> Yes, I do. And I think that we can look around the world or even to local health departments where there was a consistent, coordinated messaging helped to build trust and cooperation…. But the divisiveness early on, I think, was a major challenge. And so, you know, I do share the sentiment of this.[381]

Echoing Dr. Schuchat, Dr. Cetron stated that more Americans would be alive today if the Trump Administration had allowed CDC to provide the clear messaging and accurate guidance that public health experts were consistently calling for:

> [T]he general principles of being very up front in conveying the scientific information to the power of these nonpharmaceutical mitigations and how they

can shape the experience of this pandemic in terms of suffering and death, you know, was—is clearly—was lacking, you know. And I think that hurt. That hurt all of us. It hurts all of us and our families. And there are people, you know, who are no longer with us that would have benefited from that kind of very clear messaging.[382]

The Trump Administration's interference in CDC's efforts to respond to the pandemic and attacks against CDC scientists reflected a larger pattern of hostility that ultimately impacted a broad swath of public health officials and agencies. As the Select Subcommittee's investigations have previously revealed, the Trump White House blocked Dr. Birx from conducting national press appearances and repeatedly attacked and attempted to discredit Dr. Anthony Fauci, Director of the National Institute of Allergy and Infectious Diseases, for providing truthful information to the public that contradicted White House talking points.[383] Trump White House officials took steps to alter and suppress the weekly Governors' Reports sent by Dr. Birx to state and local officials, including weakening and deleting proposed mitigation measures and other science-based recommendations.[384] Trump White House officials executed coordinated pressure campaigns that sought to bend FDA's coronavirus decision making to the White House's political will, including pressuring the agency to reauthorize hydroxychloroquine after it was shown to be ineffective and potentially dangerous; strongarming FDA to deliver misleadingly positive news about convalescent plasma as a coronavirus treatment on the eve of the 2020 Republican National Convention; and blocking FDA from issuing guidance on coronavirus vaccine authorizations for weeks in an attempt to ensure that the first vaccine could be authorized before the 2020 presidential election.[385]

The disastrous consequences of Trump Administration officials' rampant political interference in the nation's pandemic response continue to be felt today. Public trust in medical scientists is lower now than it was before the pandemic,[386] while only 44 percent of Americans say they trust CDC's messaging about the coronavirus—down from nearly 70 percent at the outset of the pandemic.[387] Meanwhile, more than three-quarters of U.S. adults indicated that they believe or are unsure about the accuracy of at least one common false statement about the coronavirus—the end result of a deluge of pandemic misinformation pushed by faux experts and cynical profiteers, who are increasingly drowning out sound public health guidance.[388]

To adequately respond to future public health threats, Americans' faith in our public health agencies must continue to be restored. We must also continue to safeguard the independence of those institutions to ensure that the work of public health officials and experts are protected from individuals more concerned with their political ambition than Americans' wellbeing.

[1] Majority Staff, Select Subcommittee on the Coronavirus Crisis, *The Atlas Dogma: The Trump Administration's Embrace of a Dangerous and Discredited Herd Immunity via Mass Infection Strategy* (June 2022) (online at https://coronavirus.house.gov/sites/democrats.coronavirus.house.gov/files/2022.06.21%20The%20Trump%20Admi nistration%E2%80%99s%20Embrace%20of%20a%20Dangerous%20and%20Discredited%20Herd%20Immunity% 20via%20Mass%20Infection%20Strategy.pdf); Majority Staff, Select Subcommittee on the Coronavirus Crisis, *A "Knife Fight" with the FDA: The Trump White House's Relentless Attacks on FDA's Coronavirus Response* (Aug. 2020) (online at https://coronavirus.house.gov/sites/democrats.coronavirus.house.gov/files/2022.08.24%20The%20Trump%20White %20House%E2%80%99s%20Relentless%20Attacks%20on%20FDA%E2%80%99s%20Coronavirus%20Response. pdf).

[2] Centers for Disease Control and Prevention, *2020 News Releases* (online at www.cdc.gov/media/releases/2020/archives.html) (accessed on Oct. 12, 2022).

[3] Centers for Disease Control and Prevention, *Press Release: Transcript for the CDC Telebriefing Updated on COVID-19* (Feb. 26, 2020) (online at www.cdc.gov/media/releases/2020/t0225-cdc-telebriefing-covid-19.html).

[4] Select Subcommittee on the Coronavirus Crisis, Transcribed Interview of Jay Butler (Nov. 30, 2021) (online at https://coronavirus.house.gov/sites/democrats.coronavirus.house.gov/files/2021.11.30%20SSCC%20Interview%20o f%20Jay%20Butler%20-%20REDACTED.pdf).

[5] Centers for Disease Control and Prevention, *Press Release: CDC Confirms Possible Instance of Community Spread of COVID-19 in U.S.* (Feb. 26, 2020) (online at www.cdc.gov/media/releases/2020/s0226-Covid-19-spread.html).

[6] *Dow Drops More than 800 Points on CDC Warnings of Coronavirus Spread in U.S.*, CBS News (Feb. 25, 2020) (online at www.cbsnews.com/news/stocks-down-dow-plunges-after-mondays-rout-on-coronavirus-fears); *Trump Is Reportedly Furious that the Stock Market Is Plunging on Coronavirus Fears*, CNBC (Feb. 25, 2020) (online at https://cnbc.com/2020/02/25/trump-is-reportedly-furious-with-the-plunging-stock-market-due-to-coronavirus-fears.html).

[7] Select Subcommittee on the Coronavirus Crisis, Transcribed Interview of Nancy Messonnier (Oct. 8, 2021) (online at https://coronavirus.house.gov/sites/democrats.coronavirus.house.gov/files/2021.10.08%20SSCC%20Interview%20o f%20Nancy%20Messonnier%20-%20REDACTED.pdf).

[8] Select Subcommittee on the Coronavirus Crisis, Transcribed Interview of Anne Schuchat (Oct. 1, 2021) (online at https://coronavirus.house.gov/sites/democrats.coronavirus.house.gov/files/2021.10.01%20SSCC%20Interview%20o f%20Anne%20Schuchat%20-%20REDACTED.pdf).

[9] *Health Officials Warn Americans to Plan for the Spread of Coronavirus in U.S.* (Feb. 25, 2020) (online at www.npr.org/sections/health-shots/2020/02/25/809318447/health-officials-warn-americans-to-start-planning-for-spread-of-coronavirus-in-u); Department of Health and Human Services, *Health and Human Services Briefing on the Coronavirus Outbreak* (Feb. 25, 2020) (online at www.c-span.org/video/?469708-1/hhs-officials-hold-news-conference-coronavirus).

[10] Select Subcommittee on the Coronavirus Crisis, Transcribed Interview of Anne Schuchat (Oct. 1, 2021) (online at https://coronavirus.house.gov/sites/democrats.coronavirus.house.gov/files/2021.10.01%20SSCC%20Interview%20o f%20Anne%20Schuchat%20-%20REDACTED.pdf).

[11] *White House Struggles to Contain Public Alarm over Coronavirus*, Washington Post (Feb. 26, 2020) (online at www.washingtonpost.com/business/2020/02/25/white-house-struggles-contain-public-alarm-over-coronavirus-despite-panic); *Larry Kudlow Says US Has Contained the Coronavirus and the Economy Is Holding up Nicely*, CNBC (Feb. 25. 2020) (online at www.cnbc.com/2020/02/25/larry-kudlow-says-us-has-contained-the-

coronavirus-and-the-economy-is-holding-up-nicely.html); *Media's Coronavirus Stories Trying to Hurt Trump, Mick Mulvaney Says as He Urges Public to Turn off TV*, CNBC (Feb. 28, 2020) (online at https://cnbc.com/2020/02/28/trump-chief-of-staff-mulvaney-suggests-people-ignore-coronavirus-news-to-calm-markets.html).

[12] Select Subcommittee on the Coronavirus Crisis, Transcribed Interview of Nancy Messonnier (Oct. 8, 2021) (online at https://coronavirus.house.gov/sites/democrats.coronavirus.house.gov/files/2021.10.08%20SSCC%20Interview%20of%20Nancy%20Messonnier%20-%20REDACTED.pdf). During a transcribed interview with the Select Subcommittee, counsel for HHS instructed Dr. Messonnier not to provide any details regarding the substance of what she discussed with Secretary Azar or Dr. Redfield during these calls on the grounds of privilege.

[13] The White House, *Remarks by President Trump, Vice President Pence, and Members of the Coronavirus Task Force in Press Conference* (Feb. 27, 2020) (online at https://trumpwhitehouse.archives.gov/briefings-statements/remarks-president-trump-vice-president-pence-members-coronavirus-task-force-press-conference/).

[14] Select Subcommittee on the Coronavirus Crisis, Transcribed Interview of Bill Hall (Aug. 31, 2021) (online at https://coronavirus.house.gov/sites/democrats.coronavirus.house.gov/files/2021.08.31%20SSCC%20Interview%20of%20Bill%20Hall%20-%20REDACTED.pdf).

[15] *Id.*

[16] *Pence's Office Placed in Charge of Coronavirus Messaging*, CNN (Feb. 28, 2020) (online at www.cnn.com/2020/02/27/politics/pence-messaging-coronavirus/index.html).

[17] Select Subcommittee on the Coronavirus Crisis, Transcribed Interview of Kate Galatas (Sept. 30, 2021) (online at https://coronavirus.house.gov/sites/democrats.coronavirus.house.gov/files/2021.09.31%20SSCC%20Interview%20of%20Kate%20Galatas%20-%20REDACTED.pdf).

[18] *See, e.g.*, Select Subcommittee on the Coronavirus Crisis, Transcribed Interview of Anne Schuchat (Oct. 1, 2021) (online at https://coronavirus.house.gov/sites/democrats.coronavirus.house.gov/files/2021.10.01%20SSCC%20Interview%20of%20Anne%20Schuchat%20-%20REDACTED.pdf); Select Subcommittee on the Coronavirus Crisis, Transcribed Interview of Daniel Jernigan (Dec. 13, 2021) (online at https://coronavirus.house.gov/sites/democrats.coronavirus.house.gov/files/2021.12.13%20SSCC%20Interview%20of%20Daniel%20Jernigan%20-%20REDACTED.pdf).

[19] Select Subcommittee on the Coronavirus Crisis, Transcribed Interview of Daniel Jernigan (Dec. 13, 2021) (online at https://coronavirus.house.gov/sites/democrats.coronavirus.house.gov/files/2021.12.13%20SSCC%20Interview%20of%20Daniel%20Jernigan%20-%20REDACTED.pdf).

[20] Select Subcommittee on the Coronavirus Crisis, Transcribed Interview of Kate Galatas (Sept. 30, 2021) (online at https://coronavirus.house.gov/sites/democrats.coronavirus.house.gov/files/2021.09.31%20SSCC%20Interview%20of%20Kate%20Galatas%20-%20REDACTED.pdf).

[21] *See supra* Section I.A.

[22] Select Subcommittee on the Coronavirus Crisis, Transcribed Interview of Robert Redfield (Mar. 17, 2022) (online at https://coronavirus.house.gov/sites/democrats.coronavirus.house.gov/files/2022.03.17%20SSCC%20Interview%20of%20Robert%20Redfield%20-%20REDACTED.pdf).

[23] *Id.*

[24] Email from Ryan Murphy, Principal Deputy Assistant Secretary for Public Affairs, Department of Health and Human Services, to Michael Caputo, Assistant Secretary for Public Affairs, Department of Health and Human Services, et al. (May 22, 2020) (SSCC-0013702 – 03) (online at

https://coronavirus.house.gov/sites/democrats.coronavirus.house.gov/files/2020.05.22%20SSCC-0013702-05_Redacted.pdf).

[25] Centers for Disease Control and Prevention, *2020 News Releases* (online at www.cdc.gov/media/releases/2020/archives.html) (accessed on Oct. 12, 2022).

[26] Letter from Chairman James E. Clyburn, Select Subcommittee on the Coronavirus Crisis, to Robert Redfield (Nov. 12, 2021) (online at https://coronavirus.house.gov/sites/democrats.coronavirus.house.gov/files/2021-11-12%20Clyburn%20to%20Redfield_0.pdf).

[27] Select Subcommittee on the Coronavirus Crisis, Transcribed Interview of Kate Galatas (Sept. 30, 2021) (online at https://coronavirus.house.gov/sites/democrats.coronavirus.house.gov/files/2021.09.31%20SSCC%20Interview%20of%20Kate%20Galatas%20-%20REDACTED.pdf).

[28] *Id.*

[29] Select Subcommittee on the Coronavirus Crisis, Transcribed Interview of Anne Schuchat (Oct. 1, 2021) (online at https://coronavirus.house.gov/sites/democrats.coronavirus.house.gov/files/2021.10.01%20SSCC%20Interview%20of%20Anne%20Schuchat%20-%20REDACTED.pdf).

[30] *Id.*

[31] Centers for Disease Control and Prevention, *Telebriefing on Investigation of Human Cases of H1N1 Flu* (May 11, 2009) (online at www.cdc.gov/media/pressrel/2009/a090511.htm); Centers for Disease Control and Prevention, *Telebriefing - Update on Zika Pregnancy Outcomes in U.S. Territories* (June 8, 2017) (online at www.cdc.gov/media/releases/2017/t0609-zika-pregnancy-outcomes.html); Centers for Disease Control and Prevention, *Telebriefing: Measles in the United States* (Jan. 29, 2015) (online at www.cdc.gov/media/releases/2015/t0129-measles.html); Centers for Disease Control and Prevention, *Telebriefing Update on Respiratory Illness Affecting Children in Multiple States* (Sept. 8, 2014) (online at www.cdc.gov/media/releases/2014/t0908-respiratory-Illness.html).

[32] Select Subcommittee on the Coronavirus Crisis, Transcribed Interview of Anne Schuchat (Oct. 1, 2021) (online at https://coronavirus.house.gov/sites/democrats.coronavirus.house.gov/files/2021.10.01%20SSCC%20Interview%20of%20Anne%20Schuchat%20-%20REDACTED.pdf).

[33] Select Subcommittee on the Coronavirus Crisis, Transcribed Interview of Kate Galatas (Sept. 30, 2021) (online at https://coronavirus.house.gov/sites/democrats.coronavirus.house.gov/files/2021.09.31%20SSCC%20Interview%20of%20Kate%20Galatas%20-%20REDACTED.pdf).

[34] *Id.*

[35] *'We've Been Muzzled': CDC Sources Say White House Putting Politics Ahead of Science*, CNN (May 20, 2020) (online at www.cnn.com/2020/05/20/politics/coronavirus-travel-alert-cdc-white-house-tensions-invs/index.html).

[36] Email from Loretta Lepore, Senior Advisor to the Director, Centers for Disease Control and Prevention, to Robert Redfield, Director, Centers for Disease Control and Prevention, et al. (June 11, 2020) (SSCC-0038857 – 62) (online at https://coronavirus.house.gov/sites/democrats.coronavirus.house.gov/files/2020.06.11%20SSCC-0038857_Redacted.pdf).

[37] Select Subcommittee on the Coronavirus Crisis, Transcribed Interview of Anne Schuchat (Oct. 1, 2021) (online at https://coronavirus.house.gov/sites/democrats.coronavirus.house.gov/files/2021.10.01%20SSCC%20Interview%20of%20Anne%20Schuchat%20-%20REDACTED.pdf).

[38] Select Subcommittee on the Coronavirus Crisis, Transcribed Interview of Kate Galatas (Sept. 30, 2021) (online at https://coronavirus.house.gov/sites/democrats.coronavirus.house.gov/files/2021.09.31%20SSCC%20Interview%20of%20Kate%20Galatas%20-%20REDACTED.pdf).

[39] *See, e.g., 9 Controversial Moments that Led Trump to Stop His White House Coronavirus Briefings*, ABC News (Jul. 21, 2020) (online at https://abcnews.go.com/Politics/controversial-moments-led-trump-stop-white-house-coronavirus/story?id=71899110).

[40] *President Trump Says Americans Should Cover Their Mouths in Public — But He Won't*, TIME (Apr. 3, 2020) (online at https://time.com/5815615/trump-coronavirus-mixed-messaging/).

[41] Select Subcommittee on the Coronavirus Crisis, Transcribed Interview of Jay Butler (Nov. 30, 2021) (online at https://coronavirus.house.gov/sites/democrats.coronavirus.house.gov/files/2021.11.30%20SSCC%20Interview%20of%20Jay%20Butler%20-%20REDACTED.pdf).

[42] Select Subcommittee on the Coronavirus Crisis, Transcribed Interview of Anne Schuchat (Oct. 1, 2021) (online at https://coronavirus.house.gov/sites/democrats.coronavirus.house.gov/files/2021.10.01%20SSCC%20Interview%20of%20Anne%20Schuchat%20-%20REDACTED.pdf).

[43] The White House, *Remarks by President Trump, Vice President Pence, and Members of the Coronavirus Task Force in Press Conference* (Apr. 23, 2020) (online at https://trumpwhitehouse.archives.gov/briefings-statements/remarks-president-trump-vice-president-pence-members-coronavirus-task-force-press-briefing-31/); Select Subcommittee on the Coronavirus Crisis, *A Hearing with Trump White House Coronavirus Response Coordinator Dr. Deborah Birx* (June 23, 2022) (online at https://coronavirus.house.gov/subcommittee-activity/hearings/hearing-trump-white-house-coronavirus-response-coordinator-dr-deborah).

[44] Department of Homeland Security, Science and Technology Directorate, *SARS-CoV-2 Applied Research Response* (Apr. 20, 2020) (SSCC-P011396 – 400) (online at https://coronavirus.house.gov/sites/democrats.coronavirus.house.gov/files/2020.04.20%20P011396-400%20-%20NR.pdf) (emphasis added).

[45] *'It's Irresponsible and It's Dangerous': Experts Rip Trump's Idea of Injecting Disinfectant to Treat COVID-19*, NBC News (Apr. 23, 2020) (online at www.nbcnews.com/politics/donald-trump/it-s-irresponsible-it-s-dangerous-experts-rip-trump-s-n1191246); The White House, *Remarks by President Trump, Vice President Pence, and Members of the Coronavirus Task Force in Press Conference* (Apr. 23, 2020) (online at https://trumpwhitehouse.archives.gov/briefings-statements/remarks-president-trump-vice-president-pence-members-coronavirus-task-force-press-briefing-31/).

[46] *See, e.g., Accidental Poisonings Increased After President Trump's Disinfectant Comments*, TIME (May 12, 2020) (online at https://time.com/5835244/accidental-poisonings-trump/).

[47] Select Subcommittee on the Coronavirus Crisis, Transcribed Interview of Nancy Messonnier (Oct. 8, 2021) (online at https://coronavirus.house.gov/sites/democrats.coronavirus.house.gov/files/2021.10.08%20SSCC%20Interview%20of%20Nancy%20Messonnier%20-%20REDACTED.pdf); *see also* Select Subcommittee on the Coronavirus Crisis, Transcribed Interview of Kate Galatas (Sept. 30, 2021) (online at https://coronavirus.house.gov/sites/democrats.coronavirus.house.gov/files/2021.09.31%20SSCC%20Interview%20of%20Kate%20Galatas%20-%20REDACTED.pdf).

[48] Select Subcommittee on the Coronavirus Crisis, Transcribed Interview of Anne Schuchat (Oct. 1, 2021) (online at https://coronavirus.house.gov/sites/democrats.coronavirus.house.gov/files/2021.10.01%20SSCC%20Interview%20of%20Anne%20Schuchat%20-%20REDACTED.pdf).

[49] *Trump Health Official Apologizes for Facebook Outburst*, New York Times (Sept. 15, 2020) (online at www.nytimes.com/2020/09/15/us/michael-caputo-coronavirus.html); *Trump Officials Interfered with CDC Reports on Covid-19*, Politico (Sept. 11, 2020) (online at www.politico.com/news/2020/09/11/exclusive-trump-officials-interfered-with-cdc-reports-on-covid-19-412809).

[50] *White House Snubs Azar, Installs Trump Loyalist Michael Caputo as HHS Spokesperson*, Politico (Apr. 15, 2020) (online at www.politico.com/news/2020/04/15/michael-caputo-azar-hhs-189046).

[51] Select Subcommittee on the Coronavirus Crisis, Transcribed Interview of Kate Galatas (Sept. 30, 2021) (online at

https://coronavirus.house.gov/sites/democrats.coronavirus.house.gov/files/2021.09.31%20SSCC%20Interview%20of%20Kate%20Galatas%20-%20REDACTED.pdf).

[52] Letter from Chairman James E. Clyburn, Select Subcommittee on the Coronavirus Crisis, to Paul Alexander, Assistant Professor, McMaster University (Apr. 9, 2021) (online at https://coronavirus.house.gov/sites/democrats.coronavirus.house.gov/files/2021-04-08.Clyburn%20to%20Alexander%20re%20COVID%20Response%20.pdf); Majority Staff, Select Subcommittee on the Coronavirus Crisis, *The Atlas Dogma: The Trump Administration's Embrace of a Dangerous and Discredited Herd Immunity via Mass Infection Strategy* (June 2022) (online at https://coronavirus.house.gov/sites/democrats.coronavirus.house.gov/files/2022.06.21%20The%20Trump%20Administration%E2%80%99s%20Embrace%20of%20a%20Dangerous%20and%20Discredited%20Herd%20Immunity%20via%20Mass%20Infection%20Strategy.pdf).

[53] Letter from Chairman James E. Clyburn, Select Subcommittee on the Coronavirus Crisis, to Secretary of Health and Human Services Alex Azar II and Robert Redfield, Director, Centers for Disease Control and Prevention (Dec. 21, 2020) (online at https://coronavirus.house.gov/sites/democrats.coronavirus.house.gov/files/2020-12-21.Clyburn%20to%20Redfield%20and%20Azar%20re%20Subpoena%20FINAL%20_0.pdf); *see also Emails Detail Effort to Silence C.D.C. and Question Its Science*, New York Times (Sept. 18, 2020) (online at www.nytimes.com/2020/09/18/us/politics/trump-cdc-coronavirus.html).

[54] Email from Communications Specialist, Centers for Disease Control and Prevention, to Kate Galatas, Deputy Director of the Office of Associate Director for Communications, Centers for Disease Control and Prevention, and Communications Specialist, Centers for Disease Control and Prevention (June 27, 2020) (SSCCManual-000186 – 89) (online at https://coronavirus.house.gov/sites/democrats.coronavirus.house.gov/files/2020.06.27%20SSCCManual-000186-89_Redacted.pdf).

[55] Select Subcommittee on the Coronavirus Crisis, Transcribed Interview of Kate Galatas (Sept. 30, 2021) (online at https://coronavirus.house.gov/sites/democrats.coronavirus.house.gov/files/2021.09.31%20SSCC%20Interview%20of%20Kate%20Galatas%20-%20REDACTED.pdf).

[56] *White House Strips CDC of Data Collection Role for COVID-19 Hospitalizations*, National Public Radio (July 15, 2020) (online at www.npr.org/sections/health-shots/2020/07/15/891351706/white-house-strips-cdc-ofdata-collection-role-for-covid-19-hospitalizations).

[57] Email from Kate Galatas, Deputy Director of the Office of Associate Director for Communications, Centers for Disease Control and Prevention, to Robert Redfield, Director, Centers for Disease Control and Prevention, et al. (July 17, 2020) (SSCCManual000190 – 95) (online at https://coronavirus.house.gov/sites/democrats.coronavirus.house.gov/files/2020.07.17%20SSCCManual-000190-95_Redacted.pdf).

[58] Letter from Chairman James E. Clyburn, Select Subcommittee on the Coronavirus Crisis, to Secretary of Health and Human Services Alex Azar II and Robert Redfield, Director, Centers for Disease Control and Prevention (Dec. 21, 2020) (online at https://coronavirus.house.gov/sites/democrats.coronavirus.house.gov/files/2020-12-21.Clyburn%20to%20Redfield%20and%20Azar%20re%20Subpoena%20FINAL%20_0.pdf); *see also* Select Subcommittee on the Coronavirus Crisis, Transcribed Interview of Kate Galatas (Sept. 30, 2021) (online at https://coronavirus.house.gov/sites/democrats.coronavirus.house.gov/files/2021.09.31%20SSCC%20Interview%20of%20Kate%20Galatas%20-%20REDACTED.pdf).

[59] Select Subcommittee on the Coronavirus Crisis, Transcribed Interview of Kate Galatas (Sept. 30, 2021) (online at https://coronavirus.house.gov/sites/democrats.coronavirus.house.gov/files/2021.09.31%20SSCC%20Interview%20of%20Kate%20Galatas%20-%20REDACTED.pdf).

[60] Centers for Disease Control and Prevention, *Transcript – CDC Media Telebriefing: Update on COVID-19* (June 12, 2020) (online at www.cdc.gov/media/releases/2020/t0612-covid-19-update.html).

[61] Select Subcommittee on the Coronavirus Crisis, Transcribed Interview of Jay Butler (Nov. 30, 2021) (online at

https://coronavirus.house.gov/sites/democrats.coronavirus.house.gov/files/2021.11.30%20SSCC%20Interview%20o f%20Jay%20Butler%20-%20REDACTED.pdf).

[62] *Id.*

[63] Email from Paul Alexander, Senior Advisor, Department of Health and Human Services, to Michael Caputo, Assistant Secretary for Public Affairs, Department of Health and Human Services (Aug. 8, 2020) (SSCC-0016509 – 12) (online at https://coronavirus.house.gov/sites/democrats.coronavirus.house.gov/files/2020.08.08%20SSCC-0016509-12_Redacted.pdf).

[64] Email from Paul Alexander, Senior Advisor, Department of Health and Human Services, to Michael Caputo, Assistant Secretary for Public Affairs, Department of Health and Human Services, et al. (July 1, 2020) (SSCC-0006774 – 78) (online at https://coronavirus.house.gov/sites/democrats.coronavirus.house.gov/files/2020.07.01%20SSCC-0006774_Redacted.pdf).

[65] Email from Michael Caputo, Assistant Secretary for Public Affairs, Department of Health and Human Services, to Paul Alexander, Senior Advisor, Department of Health and Human Services (July 1, 2020) (SSCC-0022816 – 20) (online at https://coronavirus.house.gov/sites/democrats.coronavirus.house.gov/files/2020.07.01%20SSCC-0022816-0022820_Redacted.pdf).

[66] Email from Paul Alexander, Senior Advisor, Department of Health and Human Services, to Michael Robinson, Strategic Planning, Department of Health and Human Services (May 8, 2020) (SSCC-0014755 – 57) (online at https://coronavirus.house.gov/sites/democrats.coronavirus.house.gov/files/2020.05.08%20SSCC-0014755-57_Redacted.pdf).

[67] Select Subcommittee on the Coronavirus Crisis, Transcribed Interview of Kate Galatas (Sept. 30, 2021) (online at https://coronavirus.house.gov/sites/democrats.coronavirus.house.gov/files/2021.09.31%20SSCC%20Interview%20o f%20Kate%20Galatas%20-%20REDACTED.pdf).

[68] Select Subcommittee on the Coronavirus Crisis, Transcribed Interview of Nina Witkofsky (Feb. 2, 2022) (online at https://coronavirus.house.gov/sites/democrats.coronavirus.house.gov/files/2022.02.02.SSCC%20Interview%20of%2 0Nina%20Witkofsky%20-%20REDACTED.pdf); *see also White House Puts 'Politicals' at CDC to Try to Control Info*, Associated Press (Oct. 16, 2020) (online at https://apnews.com/article/election-2020-virus-outbreak-pandemics-public-health-new-york-b279b4ead51e0871059df4c03ad8df6e).

[69] Select Subcommittee on the Coronavirus Crisis, Transcribed Interview of Kate Galatas (Sept. 30, 2021) (online at https://coronavirus.house.gov/sites/democrats.coronavirus.house.gov/files/2021.09.31%20SSCC%20Interview%20o f%20Kate%20Galatas%20-%20REDACTED.pdf).

[70] *Id.*

[71] Select Subcommittee on the Coronavirus Crisis, Transcribed Interview of Nina Witkofsky (Feb. 2, 2022) (online at https://coronavirus.house.gov/sites/democrats.coronavirus.house.gov/files/2022.02.02.SSCC%20Interview%20of%2 0Nina%20Witkofsky%20-%20REDACTED.pdf).

[72] *See, e.g.,* Email from Madeleine Hubbard, Special Assistant, Department of Health and Human Services, to Paul Alexander, Senior Advisor, Department of Health and Human Services (June 30, 2020) (SSCC-0007093 – 110) (online at https://coronavirus.house.gov/sites/democrats.coronavirus.house.gov/files/2020.06.30%20SSCC-0007093-110_Redacted.pdf); Email from Nina Witkofsky, Senior Advisor, Centers for Disease Control and Prevention, to Ryan Murphy, Principal Deputy Assistant Secretary for Public Affairs, Department of Health and Human Services, et al. (July 28, 2020) (SSCC-0003201 – 02) (online at https://coronavirus.house.gov/sites/democrats.coronavirus.house.gov/files/2020.07.28%20SSCC-0003201-02_Redacted.pdf).

[73] Email from Paul Alexander, Senior Advisor, Department of Health and Human Services, to Michael Caputo, Assistant Secretary for Public Affairs, Department of Health and Human Services (May 8, 2020) (SSCC-0014762) (online at https://coronavirus.house.gov/sites/democrats.coronavirus.house.gov/files/2020.05.08%20SSCC-0014762%20-%2065_Redacted.pdf).

[74] Email from Paul Alexander, Senior Advisor, Department of Health and Human Services, to Benjamin Haynes, Deputy Chief, News Media Branch, Centers for Disease Control and Prevention (May 8, 2020) (SSCC-0014485) (online at https://coronavirus.house.gov/sites/democrats.coronavirus.house.gov/files/2020.05.09%20SSCC-0014485%20-%2087_Redacted.pdf). While children and young adults may, on the whole, have lesser susceptibility to severe coronavirus outcomes, the risk of severe side illness and death is not 0%. *See* Centers for Disease Control and Prevention, *Hospitalization and Death by Race/Ethnicity* (online at www.cdc.gov/coronavirus/2019-ncov/covid-data/investigations-discovery/hospitalization-death-by-race-ethnicity.html) (accessed on Oct. 14, 2022); Centers for Disease Control and Prevention, *Hospitalization and Death by Age* (online at www.cdc.gov/coronavirus/2019-ncov/covid-data/investigations-discovery/hospitalization-death-by-age.html) (accessed on Oct. 14, 2022); *Coronavirus and COVID-19: Younger Adults Are at Risk, Too*, Johns Hopkins Medicine (Dec. 2, 2020) (online at www.hopkinsmedicine.org/health/conditions-and-diseases/coronavirus/coronavirus-and-covid-19-younger-adults-are-at-risk-too).

[75] Email from Paul Alexander, Senior Advisor, Department of Health and Human Services, to Michael Caputo, Assistant Secretary for Public Affairs, Department of Health and Human Services (May 9, 2020) (SSCC-0014485) (online at https://coronavirus.house.gov/sites/democrats.coronavirus.house.gov/files/2020.05.09%20SSCC-0014485%20-%2087_Redacted.pdf).

[76] Email from Paul Alexander, Senior Advisor, Department of Health and Human Services, to Brad Traverse, Senior Advisor, Department of Health and Human Services, et al. (May 19, 2020) (SSCC-0009073) (online at https://coronavirus.house.gov/sites/democrats.coronavirus.house.gov/files/2020.05.19%20SSCC-0009073-74_Redacted.pdf).

[77] Email from Paul Alexander, Senior Advisor, Department of Health and Human Services, to Michael Robinson, Strategic Planning, Department of Health and Human Services, et al. (May 28, 2020) (SSCC-0013519 – 23) (online at https://coronavirus.house.gov/sites/democrats.coronavirus.house.gov/files/2020.05.28%20SSCC-0013519-23_Redacted.pdf).

[78] Email from Paul Alexander, Senior Advisor, Department of Health and Human Services, to Scott Pauley, Press Officer, Centers for Disease Control and Prevention, et al. (May 30, 2020) (SSCC-0009080) (online at https://coronavirus.house.gov/sites/democrats.coronavirus.house.gov/files/2020.05.30%20SSCC-0009080-83_Redacted.pdf).

[79] Email from Paul Alexander, Senior Advisor, Department of Health and Human Services, to Michael Caputo, Assistant Secretary for Public Affairs, Department of Health and Human Services, et al. (June 15, 2020) (SSCC-0007320 – 21) (online at https://coronavirus.house.gov/sites/democrats.coronavirus.house.gov/files/2020.06.15%20SSCC-007320-21_Redacted.pdf).

[80] Email from Paul Alexander, Senior Advisor, Department of Health and Human Services, to Michael Caputo, Assistant Secretary for Public Affairs, Department of Health and Human Services, et al. (June 20, 2020) (SSCCManual-000216 – 19) (online at https://coronavirus.house.gov/sites/democrats.coronavirus.house.gov/files/2020.06.20%20SSCCManual-000216%20%E2%80%93%2019_Redacted.pdf); *see also* Email from Paul Alexander, Senior Advisor, Department of Health and Human Services, to Benjamin Haynes, Deputy Chief, News Media Branch, Centers for Disease Control and Prevention, et al. (June 20, 2020) (SSCCManual-000220 – 23) (online at https://coronavirus.house.gov/sites/democrats.coronavirus.house.gov/files/2020.06.20%20SSCCManual-000220%20%E2%80%93%2023_Redacted.pdf).

[81] Email from Paul Alexander, Senior Advisor, Department of Health and Human Services, to Michael Caputo, Assistant Secretary for Public Affairs, Department of Health and Human Services, et al. (June 24, 2020) (SSCC-0007182) (online at

https://coronavirus.house.gov/sites/democrats.coronavirus.house.gov/files/2020.06.24%20SSCC-0007182_Redacted.pdf).

[82] *See, e.g.*, Select Subcommittee on the Coronavirus Crisis, Transcribed Interview of Jay Butler (Nov. 30, 2021) (online at https://coronavirus.house.gov/sites/democrats.coronavirus.house.gov/files/2021.11.30%20SSCC%20Interview%20of%20Jay%20Butler%20-%20REDACTED.pdf); Select Subcommittee on the Coronavirus Crisis, Transcribed Interview of Henry Walke (Feb. 18, 2022) (online at https://coronavirus.house.gov/sites/democrats.coronavirus.house.gov/files/2022.02.18%20SSCC%20Interview%20of%20Henry%20Walke%2C%20M.D.%20-%20REDACTED.pdf); Select Subcommittee on the Coronavirus Crisis, Transcribed Interview of Robert Redfield (Mar. 17, 2022) (online at https://coronavirus.house.gov/sites/democrats.coronavirus.house.gov/files/2022.03.17%20SSCC%20Interview%20of%20Robert%20Redfield%20-%20REDACTED.pdf); Select Subcommittee on the Coronavirus Crisis, Transcribed Interview of Anne Schuchat (Oct. 1, 2021) (online at https://coronavirus.house.gov/sites/democrats.coronavirus.house.gov/files/2021.10.01%20SSCC%20Interview%20of%20Anne%20Schuchat%20-%20REDACTED.pdf).

[83] Select Subcommittee on the Coronavirus Crisis, Transcribed Interview of Anne Schuchat (Oct. 1, 2021) (online at https://coronavirus.house.gov/sites/democrats.coronavirus.house.gov/files/2021.10.01%20SSCC%20Interview%20of%20Anne%20Schuchat%20-%20REDACTED.pdf); *see also* Centers for Disease Control and Prevention, *CDC Emergency Operations Center: CDC Public Health Response Timeline* (online at www.cdc.gov/cpr/eoc/responses.htm) (accessed on Oct. 14, 2022).

[84] Select Subcommittee on the Coronavirus Crisis, Transcribed Interview of Anne Schuchat (Oct. 1, 2021) (online at https://coronavirus.house.gov/sites/democrats.coronavirus.house.gov/files/2021.10.01%20SSCC%20Interview%20of%20Anne%20Schuchat%20-%20REDACTED.pdf).

[85] *Id.*

[86] *See* Select Subcommittee on the Coronavirus Crisis, *Press Release: Select Subcommittee Releases New Findings Detailing Trump Administration's Political Interference in Early Pandemic Response* (Apr. 29, 2022) (online at https://coronavirus.house.gov/news/press-releases/select-subcommittee-releases-new-findings-detailing-trump-administration-s); Select Subcommittee on the Coronavirus Crisis, *Press Release: Clyburn Demands Answers from Redfield on Trump Administration Officials' Interference with CDC's Pandemic Response* (Nov. 12, 2021) (online at https://coronavirus.house.gov/news/press-releases/clyburn-demands-answers-redfield-trump-administration-officials-interference-cdc).

[87] Select Subcommittee on the Coronavirus Crisis, Transcribed Interview of Anne Schuchat (Oct. 1, 2021) (online at https://coronavirus.house.gov/sites/democrats.coronavirus.house.gov/files/2021.10.01%20SSCC%20Interview%20of%20Anne%20Schuchat%20-%20REDACTED.pdf).

[88] Select Subcommittee on the Coronavirus Crisis, Transcribed Interview of Robert Redfield (Mar. 17, 2022) (online at https://coronavirus.house.gov/sites/democrats.coronavirus.house.gov/files/2022.03.17%20SSCC%20Interview%20of%20Robert%20Redfield%20-%20REDACTED.pdf).

[89] *Id.*

[90] Select Subcommittee on the Coronavirus Crisis, Transcribed Interview of Deborah Birx (Oct. 13, 2021) (online at https://coronavirus.house.gov/sites/democrats.coronavirus.house.gov/files/2021.10.13%20Birx%20TI%20Transcript%20%2B%20Errata.pdf).

[91] Centers for Disease Control and Prevention, *Overview of Testing for SARS-CoV-2* (June 13, 2020) (online at https://web.archive.org/web/20200614014804/https://www.cdc.gov/coronavirus/2019-ncov/hcp/testing-overview.html).

[92] Email from Russell Vought, Director, Office of Management and Budget, to Mark Meadows, Chief of Staff, The White House (June 18, 2020) (SSCC-0010220 – 25) (online at https://coronavirus.house.gov/sites/democrats.coronavirus.house.gov/files/2020.06.18%20OMB-SSCC-0010220-25_Redacted.pdf).

[93] Centers for Disease Control and Prevention, *Overview of Testing for SARS-CoV-2* (July 2, 2020) (online at https://web.archive.org/web/20200703034624/https:/www.cdc.gov/coronavirus/2019-ncov/hcp/testing-overview.html).

[94] Select Subcommittee on the Coronavirus Crisis, Transcribed Interview of Anne Schuchat (Oct. 1, 2021) (online at https://coronavirus.house.gov/sites/democrats.coronavirus.house.gov/files/2021.10.01%20SSCC%20Interview%20of%20Anne%20Schuchat%20-%20REDACTED.pdf).

[95] *Id.*

[96] Letter from Counsel for Kyle McGowan and Amanda Campbell to Chairman James E. Clyburn, Select Subcommittee on the Coronavirus Crisis (June 10, 2022) (online at https://coronavirus.house.gov/sites/democrats.coronavirus.house.gov/files/2022.06.10%20Letter%20to%20Chairman%20Clyburn_Redacted.pdf).

[97] Select Subcommittee on the Coronavirus Crisis, Transcribed Interview of Robert Redfield (Mar. 17, 2022) (online at https://coronavirus.house.gov/sites/democrats.coronavirus.house.gov/files/2022.03.17%20SSCC%20Interview%20of%20Robert%20Redfield%20-%20REDACTED.pdf).

[98] Select Subcommittee on the Coronavirus Crisis, Transcribed Interview of Anne Schuchat (Oct. 1, 2021) (online at https://coronavirus.house.gov/sites/democrats.coronavirus.house.gov/files/2021.10.01%20SSCC%20Interview%20of%20Anne%20Schuchat%20-%20REDACTED.pdf).

[99] *Id.*

[100] Select Subcommittee on the Coronavirus Crisis, Transcribed Interview of Robert Redfield (Mar. 17, 2022) (online at https://coronavirus.house.gov/sites/democrats.coronavirus.house.gov/files/2022.03.17%20SSCC%20Interview%20of%20Robert%20Redfield%20-%20REDACTED.pdf); *see also* Memorandum from Majority Staff to Members of the Select Subcommittee on the Coronavirus Crisis, *The Trump Administration's Pattern of Political Interference in the Nation's Coronavirus Response* (July 26, 2021) (online at https://coronavirus.house.gov/sites/democrats.coronavirus.house.gov/files/7.26.2021%20Timeline%20of%20Political%20Interference%20-%20final.pdf).

[101] Briefing by Anne Schuchat, Principal Deputy Director, Centers for Disease Control and Prevention, to Staff, Select Subcommittee on the Coronavirus Crisis (Apr. 20, 2021); Select Subcommittee on the Coronavirus Crisis, Transcribed Interview of Anne Schuchat (Oct. 1, 2021) (online at https://coronavirus.house.gov/sites/democrats.coronavirus.house.gov/files/2021.10.01%20SSCC%20Interview%20of%20Anne%20Schuchat%20-%20REDACTED.pdf); *see also* Select Subcommittee on the Coronavirus Crisis, *Press Release: Clyburn Responds to CDC Review Confirming Trump Administration Undermined Guidance as Virus Spread* (Mar. 15, 2021) (online at https://coronavirus.house.gov/news/press-releases/clyburn-responds-cdc-review-confirming-trump-administration-undermined-guidance).

[102] *See* Memorandum from Majority Staff to Members of the Select Subcommittee on the Coronavirus Crisis, *The Trump Administration's Pattern of Political Interference in the Nation's Coronavirus Response* (July 26, 2021) (online at https://coronavirus.house.gov/sites/democrats.coronavirus.house.gov/files/7.26.2021%20Timeline%20of%20Political%20Interference%20-%20final.pdf).

[103] *See* Centers for Disease Control and Prevention, *Summary of Guidance Review* (Mar. 10, 2021) (online at www.cdc.gov/coronavirus/2019-ncov/downloads/communication/Guidance-Review.pdf); Select Subcommittee on the Coronavirus Crisis, Transcribed Interview of Anne Schuchat (Oct. 1, 2021) (online at

https://coronavirus.house.gov/sites/democrats.coronavirus.house.gov/files/2021.10.01%20SSCC%20Interview%20o
f%20Anne%20Schuchat%20-%20REDACTED.pdf).

[104] *See* Majority Staff, Select Subcommittee on the Coronavirus Crisis, *"Now to Get Rid of Those Pesky Health Departments!" How the Trump Administration Helped the Meatpacking Industry Block Pandemic Worker Protections* (May 2022) (online at
https://coronavirus.house.gov/sites/democrats.coronavirus.house.gov/files/2022.5.12%20-
%20SSCC%20report%20on%20Meatpacking%20FINAL.pdf).

[105] Centers for Disease Control and Prevention, *Considerations for Restaurants and Bars* (May 18, 2020) (online at https://web.archive.org/web/20200520085535/https://www.cdc.gov/coronavirus/2019-
ncov/community/organizations/business-employers/bars-restaurants.html); Centers for Disease Control and Prevention, *Restaurants and Bars During the COVID-19 Pandemic* (online at
https://web.archive.org/web/20200515064022/https:/www.cdc.gov/coronavirus/2019-
ncov/downloads/community/restaurants-and-bars-decision-tree.pdf).

[106] Letter from Counsel for Kyle McGowan and Amanda Campbell to Chairman James E. Clyburn, Select Subcommittee on the Coronavirus Crisis (June 10, 2022) (online at
https://coronavirus.house.gov/sites/democrats.coronavirus.house.gov/files/2022.06.10%20Letter%20to%20Chairma
n%20Clyburn_Redacted.pdf).

[107] Centers for Disease Control and Prevention, *Interim Guidance for Communities of Faith* (May 23, 2020) (online at https://web.archive.org/web/20200524030747/https://www.cdc.gov/coronavirus/2019-ncov/php/faith-
based.html).

[108] *See infra* Section II.B.1.

[109] Centers for Disease Control and Prevention, *Recommendations for Election Officials and Poll Workers* (June 22, 2020) (online at https://web.archive.org/web/20200630013130/https://www.cdc.gov/coronavirus/2019-
ncov/community/election-polling-locations.html).

[110] Select Subcommittee on the Coronavirus Crisis, Transcribed Interview of Anne Schuchat (Oct. 1, 2021) (online at
https://coronavirus.house.gov/sites/democrats.coronavirus.house.gov/files/2021.10.01%20SSCC%20Interview%20o
f%20Anne%20Schuchat%20-%20REDACTED.pdf); *see also* Memorandum from Majority Staff to Members of the Select Subcommittee on the Coronavirus Crisis, *The Trump Administration's Pattern of Political Interference in the Nation's Coronavirus Response* (July 26, 2021) (online at
https://coronavirus.house.gov/sites/democrats.coronavirus.house.gov/files/7.26.2021%20Timeline%20of%20Politic
al%20Interference%20-%20final.pdf).

[111] *See* Centers for Disease Control and Prevention, *Summary of Guidance Review* (Mar. 10, 2021) (online at www.cdc.gov/coronavirus/2019-ncov/downloads/communication/Guidance-Review.pdf); Select Subcommittee on the Coronavirus Crisis, Transcribed Interview of Anne Schuchat (Oct. 1, 2021) (online at
https://coronavirus.house.gov/sites/democrats.coronavirus.house.gov/files/2021.10.01%20SSCC%20Interview%20o
f%20Anne%20Schuchat%20-%20REDACTED.pdf).

[112] See Majority Staff, Select Subcommittee on the Coronavirus Crisis, *The Atlas Dogma: The Trump Administration's Embrace of a Dangerous and Discredited Herd Immunity via Mass Infection Strategy* (June 2022) (online at
https://coronavirus.house.gov/sites/democrats.coronavirus.house.gov/files/2022.06.21%20The%20Trump%20Admi
nistration%E2%80%99s%20Embrace%20of%20a%20Dangerous%20and%20Discredited%20Herd%20Immunity%
20via%20Mass%20Infection%20Strategy.pdf).

[113] Select Subcommittee on the Coronavirus Crisis, Transcribed Interview of Anne Schuchat (Oct. 1, 2021) (online at
https://coronavirus.house.gov/sites/democrats.coronavirus.house.gov/files/2021.10.01%20SSCC%20Interview%20o
f%20Anne%20Schuchat%20-%20REDACTED.pdf); *see also* Email from Jay Butler, Coronavirus Response Incident Manager, Centers for Disease Control and Prevention, to Jennifer McQuiston, Principal Deputy Incident Manager, Centers for Disease Control and Prevention, et al. (May 24, 2020) (SSCC-0037247 – 50) (online at https://coronavirus.house.gov/sites/democrats.coronavirus.house.gov/files/2020.05.24%20SSCC-0037247-
50_Redacted.pdf).

[114] Select Subcommittee on the Coronavirus Crisis, Transcribed Interview of Jay Butler (Nov. 30, 2021) (online at https://coronavirus.house.gov/sites/democrats.coronavirus.house.gov/files/2021.11.30%20SSCC%20Interview%20of%20Jay%20Butler%20-%20REDACTED.pdf).

[115] Email from Denzel McGuire, Associate Director, Office of Management and Budget, to Russell Vought, Director, Office of Management and Budget (Apr. 18, 2020) (OMB-SSCC-0010869) (online at https://coronavirus.house.gov/sites/democrats.coronavirus.house.gov/files/2020.04.18%20OMB-SSCC-0010869-72%20-%20NR.pdf); *see also* Email from Denzel McGuire, Associate Director, Office of Management and Budget, to Russell Vought, Director, Office of Management and Budget, et al. (Apr. 18, 2020) (OMB-SSCC-0010977 – 82) (online at https://coronavirus.house.gov/sites/democrats.coronavirus.house.gov/files/2020.04.18%20OMB-SSCC-0010977-82%20-%20NR.pdf).

[116] *See* Email from Quinn Hirsch, Policy Analyst, Office of Information and Regulatory Affairs, Office of Management and Budget, to Denzel McGuire, Associate Director, Office of Management and Budget, et al. (Apr. 24, 2020) (OMB-SSCC-0010694 – 96) (online at https://coronavirus.house.gov/sites/democrats.coronavirus.house.gov/files/2020.04.25%20OMB-SSCC-0010694-96%20-%20NR.pdf).

[117] Email from Robert Redfield, Director, Centers for Disease Control and Prevention, to Olivia Troye, Homeland Security Adviser, Office of the Vice President, et al. (Apr. 24, 2020) (OMB-SSCC-0010830) (online at https://coronavirus.house.gov/sites/democrats.coronavirus.house.gov/files/2020.04.24%20OMB-SSCC-0010829-30%20-%20NR.pdf); *see also* Email from Paul Ray, Administrator, Office of Information and Regulatory Affairs, Office of Management and Budget, to Russell Vought, Director, Office of Management and Budget, and Joseph Grogan, Director, White House Domestic Policy Council (Apr. 25, 2020) (OMB-SSCC-0010694) (online at https://coronavirus.house.gov/sites/democrats.coronavirus.house.gov/files/2020.04.25%20OMB-SSCC-0010694-96%20-%20NR.pdf); Email from Paul Ray, Administrator, Office of Information and Regulatory Affairs, Office of Management and Budget, to Russell Vought, Director, Office of Management and Budget (Apr. 24, 2020) (OMB-SSCC-0010953) (online at https://coronavirus.house.gov/sites/democrats.coronavirus.house.gov/files/2020.04.24%20OMB-SSCC-0010953%20-%20NR.pdf).

[118] The Federalist Society, *Jennie Bradley Lichter, Deputy General Counsel, Catholic University of America* (online at https://fedsoc.org/contributors/jennifer-lichter) (accessed on Oct. 14, 2022).

[119] Email from Russell Vought, Director, Office of Management and Budget, to Joseph Grogan, Director, White House Domestic Policy Council, et al. (Apr. 25, 2020) (OMB-SSCC-0010694) (online at https://coronavirus.house.gov/sites/democrats.coronavirus.house.gov/files/2020.04.25%20OMB-SSCC-0010694-96%20-%20NR.pdf).

[120] Email from Paul Ray, Administrator, Office of Information and Regulatory Affairs, Office of Management and Budget, to Deborah Birx, Coronavirus Response Coordinator, The White House, et al. (Apr. 26, 2020) (OMB-SSCC-0010867) (online at https://coronavirus.house.gov/sites/democrats.coronavirus.house.gov/files/2020.04.27%20OMB-SSCC-0010867-68%20-%20NR.pdf); *see also* Email from Russell Vought, Director, Office of Management and Budget, to Marc Short, Chief of Staff to Vice President Mike Pence, The White House (Apr. 28, 2020) (OMB-SSCC-0010771) (online at https://coronavirus.house.gov/sites/democrats.coronavirus.house.gov/files/OMB-SSCC-0010771-72_Redacted.pdf) (Mr. Vought told Mr. Short that "Joe"—presumably a reference to Mr. Grogan—wanted to set up a "principals meeting" to discuss the faith communities guidance and that "the taskforce needs to have a discussion on this before we go forward"); Email from Natalie Hurst, Operation Coordinator, White House Coronavirus Task Force, to Joseph Grogan, Director, White House Domestic Policy Council, et al. (Apr. 29, 2020) (OMB-SSCC-0010917 – 19) (online at https://coronavirus.house.gov/sites/democrats.coronavirus.house.gov/files/2020.04.29%20OMB-SSCC-0010917-19%20-%20NR.pdf) (an April 29, 2020, White House Coronavirus Task Force agenda reflecting that Dr. Redfield and Director Vought were scheduled to present on updated guidance for "Places of Worship").

[121] Centers for Disease Control and Prevention, *Interim Guidance for Administrators and Leaders of Community – and Faith – Based Organizations to Plan, Prepare, and Respond to Coronavirus Disease 2019*

(Mar. 21, 2020) (online at https://web.archive.org/web/20200428001839/https://www.cdc.gov/coronavirus/2019-ncov/community/organizations/guidance-community-faith-organizations.html).

[122] Email from Katie Miller, Press Secretary, Office of the Vice President, to Derek Kan, Executive Associate Director, Office of Management and Budget, et al. (Apr. 28, 2020) (OMB-SSCC-0010836 – 37) (online at https://coronavirus.house.gov/sites/democrats.coronavirus.house.gov/files/2020.04.28%20OMB-SSCC-0010836-37%20-%20NR.pdf); *see also* Email from Katie Miller, Press Secretary, Office of the Vice President, to Jill Colvin, Associated Press (Apr. 27, 2020) (OMB-SSCC-0010927 – 29) (online at https://coronavirus.house.gov/sites/democrats.coronavirus.house.gov/files/2020.04.27%20OMB-SSCC-0010927-29_Redacted.pdf) (Ms. Miller telling a reporter that "I honestly doubt we will get this prescriptive" in the Trump Administration's coronavirus guidance).

[123] Email from Jennie Lichter, Deputy Director, White House Domestic Policy Council, to Paul Ray, Administrator, Office of Information and Regulatory Affairs, Office of Management and Budget, et al. (Apr. 30, 2020) (OMB-SSCC-0010940) (online at https://coronavirus.house.gov/sites/democrats.coronavirus.house.gov/files/2020.05.01%20OMB-SSCC-0010940-45_Redacted.pdf).

[124] Email from Marc Short, Chief of Staff, Office of the Vice President, to Russell Vought, Director, Office of Management and Budget (May 14, 2020) (OMB-SSCC-0010905 – 06) (online at https://coronavirus.house.gov/sites/democrats.coronavirus.house.gov/files/2020.05.14%20OMB-SSCC-0010905-06%20-%20NR.pdf); *CDC Releases "Decision Trees" to Help Pandemic Reopening Decisions*, CNN (May 14, 2020) (online at https://edition.cnn.com/us/live-news/us-coronavirus-update-05-14-20/h_621046cd0ac22fb4e65953265da78130); *CDC Offers Brief Checklists to Guide Businesses, Schools and Others on Reopening*, Washington Post (May 14, 2020) (online at www.washingtonpost.com/health/cdc-offers-brief-checklists-to-guide-businesses-schools-and-others-on-reopening/2020/05/14/3b46c29c-9615-11ea-91d7-cf4423d47683_story.html).

[125] Email from Jennifer McQuiston, Principal Deputy Incident Manager, Centers for Disease Control and Prevention, to Jay Butler, Coronavirus Response Incident Manager, Centers for Disease Control and Prevention (May 23, 2020) (SSCC-0037249) (online at https://coronavirus.house.gov/sites/democrats.coronavirus.house.gov/files/2020.05.24%20SSCC-0037247-50_Redacted.pdf).

[126] Select Subcommittee on the Coronavirus Crisis, Transcribed Interview of Jay Butler (Nov. 30, 2021) (online at https://coronavirus.house.gov/sites/democrats.coronavirus.house.gov/files/2021.11.30%20SSCC%20Interview%20of%20Jay%20Butler%20-%20REDACTED.pdf).

[127] Email from May Davis, Associate Counsel, The White House, to Russell Vought, Director, Office of Management and Budget, et al. (May 21, 2020) (OMB-SSCC-0010903) (online at https://coronavirus.house.gov/sites/democrats.coronavirus.house.gov/files/OMB-SSCC-0010903_Supplemental.pdf). It appears Ms. Conway also made direct edits to other pieces of reopening guidance. *See* Email from Derek Kan, Executive Associate Director, Office of Management and Budget, to Jared Kushner, Senior Advisor, The White House, et al. (Apr. 13, 2020) (OMB-0010897) (online at https://coronavirus.house.gov/sites/democrats.coronavirus.house.gov/files/2020.04.13%20OMB-0010897-99%20-%20NR.pdf).

[128] Email from May Davis, Associate Counsel, The White House, to Russell Vought, Director, Office of Management and Budget, et al. (May 21, 2020) (OMB-SSCC-0010903) (online at https://coronavirus.house.gov/sites/democrats.coronavirus.house.gov/files/OMB-SSCC-0010903_Supplemental.pdf).

[129] Email from Thomas Joannou, Strategic Advisor to the Senior Counselor, Office of Kellyanne Conway, to Kyle McGowan, Chief of Staff, Centers for Disease Control and Prevention (May 21, 2020) (OMB-SSCC-0010971) (online at https://coronavirus.house.gov/sites/democrats.coronavirus.house.gov/files/2020.05.22%20OMB-SSCC-0010968-71%20-%20NR.pdf).

[130] The White House, *Remarks by President Trump at Ford Rawsonville Components Plant* (May 21, 2020) (online at https://trumpwhitehouse.archives.gov/briefings-statements/remarks-president-trump-ford-rawsonville-components-plant/).

[131] Email from Kellyanne Conway, Counselor to the President, Executive Office of the President, to Paul Ray, Administrator, Office of Information and Regulatory Affairs, Office of Management and Budget, et al. (May 22, 2020) (OMB-SSCC-0010969) (online at https://coronavirus.house.gov/sites/democrats.coronavirus.house.gov/files/2020.05.22%20OMB-SSCC-0010968-71%20-%20NR.pdf).

[132] Email from Kellyanne Conway, Counselor to the President, Executive Office of the President, to Derek Lyons, Staff Secretary, The White House, et al. (May 22, 2020) (OMB-SSCC-0010968) (online at https://coronavirus.house.gov/sites/democrats.coronavirus.house.gov/files/2020.05.22%20OMB-SSCC-0010968-71%20-%20NR.pdf).

[133] The White House, *Press Briefings by Press Secretary Kayleigh McEnany* (May 23, 2020) (online at https://trumpwhitehouse.archives.gov/briefings-statements/press-briefing-press-secretary-kayleigh-mcenany-052220/).

[134] Select Subcommittee on the Coronavirus Crisis, Transcribed Interview of Jay Butler (Nov. 30, 2021) (online at https://coronavirus.house.gov/sites/democrats.coronavirus.house.gov/files/2021.11.30%20SSCC%20Interview%20of%20Jay%20Butler%20-%20REDACTED.pdf).

[135] Centers for Disease Control and Prevention, *Interim Guidance for Communities of Faith* (May 22, 2020) (online at https://web.archive.org/web/20200522192931/https://www.cdc.gov/coronavirus/2019-ncov/php/faith-based.html).

[136] Letter from Counsel for Kyle McGowan and Amanda Campbell to Chairman James E. Clyburn, Select Subcommittee on the Coronavirus Crisis (June 10, 2022) (online at https://coronavirus.house.gov/sites/democrats.coronavirus.house.gov/files/2022.06.10%20Letter%20to%20Chairman%20Clyburn_Redacted.pdf); Select Subcommittee on the Coronavirus Crisis, Transcribed Interview of Jay Butler (Nov. 30, 2021) (online at https://coronavirus.house.gov/sites/democrats.coronavirus.house.gov/files/2021.11.30%20SSCC%20Interview%20of%20Jay%20Butler%20-%20REDACTED.pdf). In his transcribed interview, Dr. Redfield said the CDC team working on the faith communities guidance posted the initial version "without the approval of the CDC director or the approval of Henry Walke [Incident Manager for CDC's coronavirus response]." Select Subcommittee on the Coronavirus Crisis, Transcribed Interview of Robert Redfield (Mar. 17, 2022) (online at https://coronavirus.house.gov/sites/democrats.coronavirus.house.gov/files/2022.03.17%20SSCC%20Interview%20of%20Robert%20Redfield%20-%20REDACTED.pdf).

[137] Select Subcommittee on the Coronavirus Crisis, Transcribed Interview of Jay Butler (Nov. 30, 2021) (online at https://coronavirus.house.gov/sites/democrats.coronavirus.house.gov/files/2021.11.30%20SSCC%20Interview%20of%20Jay%20Butler%20-%20REDACTED.pdf).

[138] Select Subcommittee on the Coronavirus Crisis, Transcribed Interview of Robert Redfield (Mar. 17, 2022) (online at https://coronavirus.house.gov/sites/democrats.coronavirus.house.gov/files/2022.03.17%20SSCC%20Interview%20of%20Robert%20Redfield%20-%20REDACTED.pdf).

[139] Select Subcommittee on the Coronavirus Crisis, Transcribed Interview of Anne Schuchat (Oct. 1, 2021) (online at https://coronavirus.house.gov/sites/democrats.coronavirus.house.gov/files/2021.10.01%20SSCC%20Interview%20of%20Anne%20Schuchat%20-%20REDACTED.pdf).

[140] Email from Olivia Troye, Homeland Security Adviser, Office of the Vice President, to Kellyanne Conway, Counselor to the President, Executive Office of the President, et al. (May 23, 2020) (OMB-SSCC-0010925-26) (online at https://coronavirus.house.gov/sites/democrats.coronavirus.house.gov/files/2020.05.23%20OMB-SSCC-0010925-26%20-%20NR.pdf).

[141] Select Subcommittee on the Coronavirus Crisis, Transcribed Interview of Robert Redfield (Mar. 17, 2022) (online at https://coronavirus.house.gov/sites/democrats.coronavirus.house.gov/files/2022.03.17%20SSCC%20Interview%20of%20Robert%20Redfield%20-%20REDACTED.pdf).

[142] Select Subcommittee on the Coronavirus Crisis, Transcribed Interview of Jay Butler (Nov. 30, 2021) (online at https://coronavirus.house.gov/sites/democrats.coronavirus.house.gov/files/2021.11.30%20SSCC%20Interview%20of%20Jay%20Butler%20-%20REDACTED.pdf).

[143] Email from Jay Butler, Coronavirus Response Incident Manager, Centers for Disease Control and Prevention, to Jennifer McQuiston, Principal Deputy Incident Manager, Centers for Disease Control and Prevention, et al. (May 23, 2020) (SSCC-0037247-50) (online at https://coronavirus.house.gov/sites/democrats.coronavirus.house.gov/files/2020.05.24%20SSCC-0037247-50_Redacted.pdf).

[144] *Id.*

[145] Select Subcommittee on the Coronavirus Crisis, Transcribed Interview of Jay Butler (Nov. 30, 2021) (online at https://coronavirus.house.gov/sites/democrats.coronavirus.house.gov/files/2021.11.30%20SSCC%20Interview%20of%20Jay%20Butler%20-%20REDACTED.pdf).

[146] *Id.*

[147] *See A Demoralized CDC Grapples with White House Meddling and Its Own Mistakes*, Wall Street Journal (Oct. 15, 2020) (online at https://wsj.com/articles/a-demoralized-cdc-grapples-with-white-house-meddling-and-its-own-mistakes-11602776561).

[148] Select Subcommittee on the Coronavirus Crisis, Transcribed Interview of Jay Butler (Nov. 30, 2021) (online at https://coronavirus.house.gov/sites/democrats.coronavirus.house.gov/files/2021.11.30%20SSCC%20Interview%20of%20Jay%20Butler%20-%20REDACTED.pdf).

[149] Letter from Counsel for Kyle McGowan and Amanda Campbell to Chairman James E. Clyburn, Select Subcommittee on the Coronavirus Crisis (June 10, 2022) (online at https://coronavirus.house.gov/sites/democrats.coronavirus.house.gov/files/2022.06.10%20Letter%20to%20Chairman%20Clyburn_Redacted.pdf).

[150] Centers for Disease Control and Prevention, *Restaurants and Bars During the COVID-19 Pandemic* (online at https://web.archive.org/web/20200515064022/https:/www.cdc.gov/coronavirus/2019-ncov/downloads/community/restaurants-and-bars-decision-tree.pdf) (accessed Oct. 14, 2022). CDC also released a longer guidance document that similarly encouraged industry to "Limit seating capacity to allow for social distancing," without expressly defining the term in that section of the guidance. Centers for Disease Control and Prevention, *Considerations for Restaurants and Bars* (May 18, 2020) (online at https://web.archive.org/web/20200520085535/https:/www.cdc.gov/coronavirus/2019-ncov/community/organizations/business-employers/bars-restaurants.html).

[151] Select Subcommittee on the Coronavirus Crisis, Transcribed Interview of Henry Walke (Feb. 18, 2022) (online at https://coronavirus.house.gov/sites/democrats.coronavirus.house.gov/files/2022.02.18%20SSCC%20Interview%20of%20Henry%20Walke%2C%20M.D.%20-%20REDACTED.pdf).

[152] Majority Staff, Select Subcommittee on the Coronavirus Crisis, *The Atlas Dogma: The Trump Administration's Embrace of a Dangerous and Discredited Herd Immunity via Mass Infection Strategy* (June 2022) (online at https://coronavirus.house.gov/sites/democrats.coronavirus.house.gov/files/2022.06.21%20The%20Trump%20Administration%E2%80%99s%20Embrace%20of%20a%20Dangerous%20and%20Discredited%20Herd%20Immunity%20via%20Mass%20Infection%20Strategy.pdf).

[153] Email from Deborah Birx, Coronavirus Response Coordinator, The White House, to Anthony Fauci, Director, National Institute for Allergy and Infectious Diseases, et al. (Aug. 11, 2020) (010P-R000014065_0001)

(online at https://coronavirus.house.gov/sites/democrats.coronavirus.house.gov/files/2020.08.11%20010P-R000014065_0001_Redacted.pdf); *see also* Email from Deborah Birx, Coronavirus Response Coordinator, The White House, to Seema Verma, Administrator, Centers for Medicare and Medicaid Services, et al. (Aug.13, 2020) (010P-R000014068_0001) (online at https://coronavirus.house.gov/sites/democrats.coronavirus.house.gov/files/2020.08.13%20010P-R000014068_0001-02_Redacted.pdf).

[154] Select Subcommittee on the Coronavirus Crisis, Transcribed Interview of Brett Giroir (May 3, 2022) (online at https://coronavirus.house.gov/sites/democrats.coronavirus.house.gov/files/Transcribed%20Interview%20of%20Brett%20Giroir.pdf).

[155] Majority Staff, Select Subcommittee on the Coronavirus Crisis, *The Atlas Dogma: The Trump Administration's Embrace of a Dangerous and Discredited Herd Immunity via Mass Infection Strategy* (June 2022) (online at https://coronavirus.house.gov/sites/democrats.coronavirus.house.gov/files/2022.06.21%20The%20Trump%20Administration%E2%80%99s%20Embrace%20of%20a%20Dangerous%20and%20Discredited%20Herd%20Immunity%20via%20Mass%20Infection%20Strategy.pdf).

[156] *Id.*

[157] *Id.*

[158] Select Subcommittee on the Coronavirus Crisis, Transcribed Interview of Robert Redfield (Mar. 17, 2022) (online at https://coronavirus.house.gov/sites/democrats.coronavirus.house.gov/files/2022.03.17%20SSCC%20Interview%20of%20Robert%20Redfield%20-%20REDACTED.pdf).

[159] *See* Select Subcommittee on the Coronavirus Crisis, Transcribed Interview of Martin Cetron (May 2, 2022) (online at https://coronavirus.house.gov/sites/democrats.coronavirus.house.gov/files/2022.05.02%20SSCC%20Interview%20of%20Martin%20Cetron%20-%20REDACTED.pdf); Select Subcommittee on the Coronavirus Crisis, Transcribed Interview of Anne Schuchat (Oct. 1, 2021) (online at https://coronavirus.house.gov/sites/democrats.coronavirus.house.gov/files/2021.10.01%20SSCC%20Interview%20of%20Anne%20Schuchat%20-%20REDACTED.pdf).

[160] Centers for Disease Control and Prevention, *Order Suspending Introduction of Certain Persons from Countries Where a Communicable Disease Exists* (Mar. 20, 2020) (online at https://cdc.gov/quarantine/pdf/CDC-Order-Prohibiting-Introduction-of-Persons_Final_3-20-20_3-p.pdf). Title 42 authorizes HHS to take measures to prevent the entry and spread of communicable diseases from foreign countries into the United States and between states. HHS has delegated this authority to CDC. Centers for Disease Control and Prevention, *Legal Authorities for Isolation and Quarantine* (Sept. 17, 2021) (online at https://cdc.gov/quarantine/aboutlawsregulationsquarantineisolation.html).

[161] *See, e.g.*, *Pence Ordered Borders Closed After CDC Experts Refused*, Associated Press (Oct. 3, 2020) (online at https://apnews.com/article/virus-outbreak-pandemics-public-health-new-york-health-4ef0c6c5263815a26f8aa17f6ea490ae).

[162] Select Subcommittee on the Coronavirus Crisis, Transcribed Interview of Martin Cetron (May 2, 2022) (online at https://coronavirus.house.gov/sites/democrats.coronavirus.house.gov/files/2022.05.02%20SSCC%20Interview%20of%20Martin%20Cetron%20-%20REDACTED.pdf).

[163] *Emails Show Stephen Miller Led Efforts to Expel Migrants at Border Under Title 42*, American Oversight (Mar. 21, 2022) (online at https://americanoversight.org/emails-show-stephen-miller-led-efforts-to-expel-migrants-at-the-border-under-title-42); *Inside the Fall of the CDC*, ProPublica (Oct. 15, 2020) (online at https://propublica.org/article/inside-the-fall-of-the-cdc); *How Trump Came to Enforce a Practice of Separating Migrant Families*, New York Times (June 16, 2018) (online at https://nytimes.com/2018/06/16/us/politics/family-separation-trump.html); *Meet Stephen Miller, Architect of First Travel Ban, Whose Words May Haunt Him*, The Guardian (Mar. 15, 2017) (online at https://theguardian.com/us-news/2017/mar/15/stephen-miller-new-trump-travel-ban).

[164] Select Subcommittee on the Coronavirus Crisis, Transcribed Interview of Robert Redfield (Mar. 17, 2022) (online at https://coronavirus.house.gov/sites/democrats.coronavirus.house.gov/files/2022.03.17%20SSCC%20Interview%20of%20Robert%20Redfield%20-%20REDACTED.pdf).

[165] Select Subcommittee on the Coronavirus Crisis, Transcribed Interview of Martin Cetron (May 2, 2022) (online at https://coronavirus.house.gov/sites/democrats.coronavirus.house.gov/files/2022.05.02%20SSCC%20Interview%20of%20Martin%20Cetron%20-%20REDACTED.pdf).

[166] *Id.*

[167] *Id.*

[168] Select Subcommittee on the Coronavirus Crisis, Transcribed Interview of Anne Schuchat (Oct. 1, 2021) (online at https://coronavirus.house.gov/sites/democrats.coronavirus.house.gov/files/2021.10.01%20SSCC%20Interview%20of%20Anne%20Schuchat%20-%20REDACTED.pdf).

[169] Select Subcommittee on the Coronavirus Crisis, Transcribed Interview of Martin Cetron (May 2, 2022) (online at https://coronavirus.house.gov/sites/democrats.coronavirus.house.gov/files/2022.05.02%20SSCC%20Interview%20of%20Martin%20Cetron%20-%20REDACTED.pdf).

[170] Select Subcommittee on the Coronavirus Crisis, Transcribed Interview of Robert Redfield (Mar. 17, 2022) (online at https://coronavirus.house.gov/sites/democrats.coronavirus.house.gov/files/2022.03.17%20SSCC%20Interview%20of%20Robert%20Redfield%20-%20REDACTED.pdf); Select Subcommittee on the Coronavirus Crisis, Transcribed Interview of Martin Cetron (May 2, 2022) (online at https://coronavirus.house.gov/sites/democrats.coronavirus.house.gov/files/2022.05.02%20SSCC%20Interview%20of%20Martin%20Cetron%20-%20REDACTED.pdf).

[171] *Inside the Fall of the CDC*, ProPublica (Oct. 15, 2020) (online at https://propublica.org/article/inside-the-fall-of-the-cdc).

[172] Select Subcommittee on the Coronavirus Crisis, Transcribed Interview of Martin Cetron (May 2, 2022) (online at https://coronavirus.house.gov/sites/democrats.coronavirus.house.gov/files/2022.05.02%20SSCC%20Interview%20of%20Martin%20Cetron%20-%20REDACTED.pdf).

[173] *Id.*

[174] *Id.*

[175] Select Subcommittee on the Coronavirus Crisis, Transcribed Interview of Robert Redfield (Mar. 17, 2022) (online at https://coronavirus.house.gov/sites/democrats.coronavirus.house.gov/files/2022.03.17%20SSCC%20Interview%20of%20Robert%20Redfield%20-%20REDACTED.pdf).

[176] Select Subcommittee on the Coronavirus Crisis, Transcribed Interview of Anne Schuchat (Oct. 1, 2021) (online at https://coronavirus.house.gov/sites/democrats.coronavirus.house.gov/files/2021.10.01%20SSCC%20Interview%20of%20Anne%20Schuchat%20-%20REDACTED.pdf).

[177] Select Subcommittee on the Coronavirus Crisis, Transcribed Interview of Martin Cetron (May 2, 2022) (online at https://coronavirus.house.gov/sites/democrats.coronavirus.house.gov/files/2022.05.02%20SSCC%20Interview%20of%20Martin%20Cetron%20-%20REDACTED.pdf).

[178] Select Subcommittee on the Coronavirus Crisis, Transcribed Interview of Anne Schuchat (Oct. 1, 2021) (online at https://coronavirus.house.gov/sites/democrats.coronavirus.house.gov/files/2021.10.01%20SSCC%20Interview%20of%20Anne%20Schuchat%20-%20REDACTED.pdf).

[179] Select Subcommittee on the Coronavirus Crisis, Transcribed Interview of Martin Cetron (May 2, 2022) (online at https://coronavirus.house.gov/sites/democrats.coronavirus.house.gov/files/2022.05.02%20SSCC%20Interview%20of%20Martin%20Cetron%20-%20REDACTED.pdf). In a September 12, 2020, email to Dr. Birx, Secretary Azar noted that it was "Depressing" that there was "not a mask in sight" at a soccer game he attended in Maryland. Email from Alex Azar II, Secretary, Department of Health and Human Services, to Deborah Birx, Coronavirus Response Coordinator, The White House (Sept. 12, 2020) (R013532) (online at https://coronavirus.house.gov/sites/democrats.coronavirus.house.gov/files/2020.09.12%20R013532_Redacted.pdf).

[180] Select Subcommittee on the Coronavirus Crisis, Transcribed Interview of Deborah Birx (Oct. 13, 2021), (online at https://coronavirus.house.gov/sites/democrats.coronavirus.house.gov/files/2021.10.13%20Birx%20TI%20Transcript%20%2B%20Errata.pdf).

[181] White House Coronavirus Task Force Agenda (July 31, 2020) (P011103) (online at https://coronavirus.house.gov/sites/democrats.coronavirus.house.gov/files/2020.07.31%20P011103%20-%20NR.pdf).

[182] Select Subcommittee on the Coronavirus Crisis, Transcribed Interview of Martin Cetron (May 2, 2022) (online at https://coronavirus.house.gov/sites/democrats.coronavirus.house.gov/files/2022.05.02%20SSCC%20Interview%20of%20Martin%20Cetron%20-%20REDACTED.pdf).

[183] Centers for Disease Control and Prevention, *No Sail Order and Other Measures Related to Operations* (Mar. 15, 2020) (online at https://cdc.gov/quarantine/pdf/signed-manifest-order_031520.pdf); *see also* Centers for Disease Control and Prevention, *CDC Announces Modifications and Extension of No Sail Order for All Cruise Ships* (Apr. 9, 2020) (online at https://cdc.gov/media/releases/2020/s0409-modifications-extension-no-sail-ships.html). According to CDC data, there were at least 41 coronavirus deaths on cruise ships in U.S. waters between March 1 and September 29, 2020. Centers for Disease Control and Prevention, *Cruise Ship No Sail Order Extended Through October 31, 2020* (Sept. 30, 2020) (online at https://cdc.gov/media/releases/2020/s0930-no-sail-order.html).

[184] Select Subcommittee on the Coronavirus Crisis, Transcribed Interview of Anne Schuchat (Oct. 1, 2021) (online at https://coronavirus.house.gov/sites/democrats.coronavirus.house.gov/files/2021.10.01%20SSCC%20Interview%20of%20Anne%20Schuchat%20-%20REDACTED.pdf).

[185] Select Subcommittee on the Coronavirus Crisis, Transcribed Interview of Martin Cetron (May 2, 2022) (online at https://coronavirus.house.gov/sites/democrats.coronavirus.house.gov/files/2022.05.02%20SSCC%20Interview%20of%20Martin%20Cetron%20-%20REDACTED.pdf).

[186] Centers for Disease Control and Prevention, *No Sail Order and Other Measures Related to Operations* (Mar. 15, 2020) (online at https://cdc.gov/quarantine/pdf/signed-manifest-order_031520.pdf); Select Subcommittee on the Coronavirus Crisis, Transcribed Interview of Anne Schuchat (Oct. 1, 2021) (online at https://coronavirus.house.gov/sites/democrats.coronavirus.house.gov/files/2021.10.01%20SSCC%20Interview%20of%20Anne%20Schuchat%20-%20REDACTED.pdf); Email from Martin Cetron, Director of the Division of Global Migration and Quarantine, Centers for Disease and Prevention, to Robert Redfield, Director, Centers for Disease Control and Prevention, et al. (Apr. 5, 2020) (SSCC-0040686) (online at https://coronavirus.house.gov/sites/democrats.coronavirus.house.gov/files/2020.04.05%20SSCC-0040686_Redacted.pdf); *see also Inside the Fall of the CDC*, ProPublica (Oct. 15, 2020) (online at https://propublica.org/article/inside-the-fall-of-the-cdc).

[187] Email from Martin Cetron, Director of the Division of Global Migration and Quarantine, Centers for Disease and Prevention, to Robert Redfield, Director, Centers for Disease Control and Prevention, et al. (Apr. 5, 2020) (SSCC-0040686) (online at https://coronavirus.house.gov/sites/democrats.coronavirus.house.gov/files/2020.04.05%20SSCC-0040686_Redacted.pdf).

[188] Select Subcommittee on the Coronavirus Crisis, Transcribed Interview of Martin Cetron (May 2, 2022) (online at

https://coronavirus.house.gov/sites/democrats.coronavirus.house.gov/files/2022.05.02%20SSCC%20Interview%20o
f%20Martin%20Cetron%20-%20REDACTED.pdf).

[189] White House Coronavirus Task Force Agenda (Apr. 5, 2020) (P009622) (online at
https://coronavirus.house.gov/sites/democrats.coronavirus.house.gov/files/2020.04.05%20P009622%20-
%20NR.pdf); White House Coronavirus Task Force Agenda (Apr. 7, 2020) (P009560) (online at
https://coronavirus.house.gov/sites/democrats.coronavirus.house.gov/files/2020.04.07%20P009560%20-
%20NR.pdf).

[190] Select Subcommittee on the Coronavirus Crisis, Transcribed Interview of Martin Cetron (May 2, 2022)
(online at
https://coronavirus.house.gov/sites/democrats.coronavirus.house.gov/files/2022.05.02%20SSCC%20Interview%20o
f%20Martin%20Cetron%20-%20REDACTED.pdf); *Inside the Fall of the CDC*, ProPublica (Oct. 15, 2020) (online
at https://propublica.org/article/inside-the-fall-of-the-cdc). When asked to elaborate on the disagreement that arose
during the interagency process, counsel for HHS asserted deliberative process privilege and instructed Dr. Cetron
not to answer. Select Subcommittee on the Coronavirus Crisis, Transcribed Interview of Martin Cetron (May 2,
2022) (online at
https://coronavirus.house.gov/sites/democrats.coronavirus.house.gov/files/2022.05.02%20SSCC%20Interview%20o
f%20Martin%20Cetron%20-%20REDACTED.pdf).

[191] Centers for Disease Control and Prevention, *CDC Announces Modifications and Extension of No Sail
Order for All Cruise Ships* (Apr. 9, 2020) (online at https://cdc.gov/media/releases/2020/s0409-modifications-
extension-no-sail-ships.html); Centers for Disease Control and Prevention, *No Sail Order and Suspension of Further
Embarkation; Notice of Modification and Extension and Other Measures Related to Operations*, 85 Fed. Reg. 21004
(Apr. 15, 2020) (notice).

[192] Select Subcommittee on the Coronavirus Crisis, Transcribed Interview of Martin Cetron (May 2, 2022)
(online at
https://coronavirus.house.gov/sites/democrats.coronavirus.house.gov/files/2022.05.02%20SSCC%20Interview%20o
f%20Martin%20Cetron%20-%20REDACTED.pdf).

[193] *See* Centers for Disease Control and Prevention, *Framework for Conditional Sailing and Initial Phase
COVID-19 Testing Requirements for Protection of Crew* (Oct. 30, 2020) (online at
https://cdc.gov/quarantine/pdf/CDC-Conditional-Sail-Order_10_30_2020-p.pdf) (noting the extensions and
expiration date).

[194] *See White House Blocked C.D.C. Order to Keep Cruise Ships Docked*, New York Times (Sept. 30,
2020) (online at https://nytimes.com/2020/09/30/health/covid-cruise-ships.html); *'We Want to See the Cruise Ships
Sail Again': Florida Governor Says He's Working with White House*, NBC WESH (Oct. 27, 2020) (online at
https://wesh.com/article/cruises-return-florida-governor-white-house/34497947).

[195] Select Subcommittee on the Coronavirus Crisis, Transcribed Interview of Robert Redfield (Mar. 17,
2022) (online at
https://coronavirus.house.gov/sites/democrats.coronavirus.house.gov/files/2022.03.17%20SSCC%20Interview%20o
f%20Robert%20Redfield%20-%20REDACTED.pdf); *see also White House Blocked C.D.C. Order to Keep Cruise
Ships Docked*, New York Times (Sept. 30, 2020) (online at https://nytimes.com/2020/09/30/health/covid-cruise-
ships.html).

[196] White House Coronavirus Task Force Agenda (July 15, 2020) (P002737) (online at
https://coronavirus.house.gov/sites/democrats.coronavirus.house.gov/files/2020.07.15%20P002737%20-
%20NR.pdf).

[197] Select Subcommittee on the Coronavirus Crisis, Transcribed Interview of Robert Redfield (Mar. 17,
2022) (online at
https://coronavirus.house.gov/sites/democrats.coronavirus.house.gov/files/2022.03.17%20SSCC%20Interview%20o
f%20Robert%20Redfield%20-%20REDACTED.pdf).

[198] Select Subcommittee on the Coronavirus Crisis, Transcribed Interview of Anne Schuchat (Oct. 1, 2021)
(online at
https://coronavirus.house.gov/sites/democrats.coronavirus.house.gov/files/2021.10.01%20SSCC%20Interview%20o
f%20Anne%20Schuchat%20-%20REDACTED.pdf).

[199] Select Subcommittee on the Coronavirus Crisis, Transcribed Interview of Robert Redfield (Mar. 17, 2022) (online at https://coronavirus.house.gov/sites/democrats.coronavirus.house.gov/files/2022.03.17%20SSCC%20Interview%20of%20Robert%20Redfield%20-%20REDACTED.pdf); Select Subcommittee on the Coronavirus Crisis, Transcribed Interview of Martin Cetron (May 2, 2022) (online at https://coronavirus.house.gov/sites/democrats.coronavirus.house.gov/files/2022.05.02%20SSCC%20Interview%20of%20Martin%20Cetron%20-%20REDACTED.pdf).

[200] Select Subcommittee on the Coronavirus Crisis, Transcribed Interview of Robert Redfield (Mar. 17, 2022) (online at https://coronavirus.house.gov/sites/democrats.coronavirus.house.gov/files/2022.03.17%20SSCC%20Interview%20of%20Robert%20Redfield%20-%20REDACTED.pdf).

[201] *Id.*; Centers for Disease Control and Prevention, *Framework for Conditional Sailing and Initial Phase COVID-19 Testing Requirements for Protection of Crew* (Oct. 30, 2020) (online at https://cdc.gov/quarantine/pdf/CDC-Conditional-Sail-Order_10_30_2020-p.pdf); *see* White House Coronavirus Task Force Agenda (Oct. 16, 2020) (P003137) (online at https://coronavirus.house.gov/sites/democrats.coronavirus.house.gov/files/2020.10.16%20P003137%20-%20NR.pdf) (reflecting that Dr. Redfield was scheduled to present on the Conditional Sail Order).

[202] Select Subcommittee on the Coronavirus Crisis, Transcribed Interview of Robert Redfield (Mar. 17, 2022) (online at https://coronavirus.house.gov/sites/democrats.coronavirus.house.gov/files/2022.03.17%20SSCC%20Interview%20of%20Robert%20Redfield%20-%20REDACTED.pdf).

[203] Centers for Disease Control and Prevention, *Press Release: CDC Issues Framework for Resuming Safe and Responsible Cruise Ship Passenger Operations* (Oct. 30, 2020) (online at https://cdc.gov/media/releases/2020/s1030-safe-responsible-ship-passenger-operations.html).

[204] Select Subcommittee on the Coronavirus Crisis, Transcribed Interview of Martin Cetron (May 2, 2022) (online at https://coronavirus.house.gov/sites/democrats.coronavirus.house.gov/files/2022.05.02%20SSCC%20Interview%20of%20Martin%20Cetron%20-%20REDACTED.pdf).

[205] Select Subcommittee on the Coronavirus Crisis, Transcribed Interview of Robert Redfield (Mar. 17, 2022) (online at https://coronavirus.house.gov/sites/democrats.coronavirus.house.gov/files/2022.03.17%20SSCC%20Interview%20of%20Robert%20Redfield%20-%20REDACTED.pdf).

[206] *Id.*

[207] *Id.*

[208] Select Subcommittee on the Coronavirus Crisis, Transcribed Interview of Martin Cetron (May 2, 2022) (online at https://coronavirus.house.gov/sites/democrats.coronavirus.house.gov/files/2022.05.02%20SSCC%20Interview%20of%20Martin%20Cetron%20-%20REDACTED.pdf).

[209] Email from Paul Alexander, Senior Advisor, Department of Health and Human Services, to Bill Hall, Deputy Assistant Secretary for Public Affairs, Department of Health and Human Services (May 22, 2020) (SSCC008869 – 71) (online at https://coronavirus.house.gov/sites/democrats.coronavirus.house.gov/files/2020.05.22%20SSCC-0008869-71_Redacted.pdf).

[210] Dr. Michelle A. Jorden, et al., *Evidence for Limited Early Spread of COVID-19 Within the United States, January–February 2020*, Morbidity and Mortality Weekly Report (June 5, 2020) (online at www.cdc.gov/mmwr/volumes/69/wr/mm6922e1.htm) (emphasis added).

[211] Email from Paul Alexander, Senior Advisor, Department of Health and Human Services, to Michael Caputo, Assistant Secretary for Public Affairs, Department of Health and Human Services (May 24, 2020) (SSCC-0013552 – 53) (online at

https://coronavirus.house.gov/sites/democrats.coronavirus.house.gov/files/2020.05.24%20SSCC-0013552_Redacted.pdf).

[212] Email from Robert Redfield, Director, Centers for Disease Control and Prevention, to Michael Caputo, Assistant Secretary for Public Affairs, Department of Health and Human Services, et al. (May 24, 2020) (SSCC-0035833-34) (online at https://coronavirus.house.gov/sites/democrats.coronavirus.house.gov/files/2020.05.24%20SSCC-0035833-34_Redacted.pdf); Email from Paul Alexander, Senior Advisor, Department of Health and Human Services, to Michael Caputo, Assistant Secretary for Public Affairs, Department of Health and Human Services (May 24, 2020) (SSCC-0035835-50) (online at https://coronavirus.house.gov/sites/democrats.coronavirus.house.gov/files/2020.05.24%20SSCC-0035835-50_Redacted.pdf).

[213] Email from Paul Alexander, Senior Advisor, Department of Health and Human Services, to Michael Caputo, Assistant Secretary for Public Affairs, Department of Health and Human Services (May 25, 2020) (SSCC-0022064-68) (online at https://coronavirus.house.gov/sites/democrats.coronavirus.house.gov/files/2020.05.25%20SSCC-0022064-68_Redacted.pdf); Email from Paul Alexander, Senior Advisor, Department of Health and Human Services, to Michael Caputo, Assistant Secretary for Public Affairs, Department of Health and Human Services, et al. (May 25, 2020) (SSCC-0014251) (online at https://coronavirus.house.gov/sites/democrats.coronavirus.house.gov/files/2020.05.25%20SSCC-0014251-62_Redacted.pdf).

[214] Email from Robert Redfield, Director, Centers for Disease Control and Prevention, to Kyle McGowan, Chief of Staff, Centers for Disease Control and Prevention (May 21, 2020) (SSCC-0018392 – 95) (online at https://coronavirus.house.gov/sites/democrats.coronavirus.house.gov/files/2020.05.22%20SSCC-0018392-95_Redacted.pdf); Appointment from Teresa Williams, Centers for Disease Control and Prevention, to Robert Redfield, Director, Centers for Disease Control and Prevention, et al. (May 22, 2020) (SSCC-0021435) (online at https://coronavirus.house.gov/sites/democrats.coronavirus.house.gov/files/2020.05.22%20SSCC-0021435_Redacted.pdf).

[215] Email from Robert Redfield, Director, Centers for Disease Control and Prevention, to Kyle McGowan, Chief of Staff, Centers for Disease Control and Prevention (May 21, 2020) (SSCC-0018392 – 95) (online at https://coronavirus.house.gov/sites/democrats.coronavirus.house.gov/files/2020.05.22%20SSCC-0018392-95_Redacted.pdf).

[216] Dr. Michelle A. Jorden, et al., *Evidence for Limited Early Spread of COVID-19 Within the United States, January–February 2020*, Morbidity and Mortality Weekly Report (June 5, 2020) (online at www.cdc.gov/mmwr/volumes/69/wr/mm6922e1.htm).

[217] Email from Paul Alexander, Senior Advisor, Department of Health and Human Services, to Michael Caputo, Assistant Secretary for Public Affairs, Department of Health and Human Services, et al. (May 14, 2022) (SSCC-0014579 – 81) (online at https://coronavirus.house.gov/sites/democrats.coronavirus.house.gov/files/2020.05.14%20SSCC-0014579-81_Redacted.pdf); *see also* Email from Paul Alexander, Senior Advisor, Department of Health and Human Services, to Bill Hall, Deputy Assistant Secretary for Public Affairs, Department of Health and Human Services, et al. (May 13, 2020) (SSCC-0014555 – 60) (online at https://coronavirus.house.gov/sites/democrats.coronavirus.house.gov/files/2020.05.14%20SSCC-0014555-60_Redacted.pdf).

[218] Centers for Disease Control and Prevention, *Emergency Preparedness and Response: Health Alert Network (HAN)* (online at https://emergency.cdc.gov/han/) (accessed Sept. 29, 2022).

[219] Email from Paul Alexander, Senior Advisor, Department of Health and Human Services, to Michael Caputo, Assistant Secretary for Public Affairs, Department of Health and Human Services (May 14, 2020) (SSCC-0014393 – 96) (online at https://coronavirus.house.gov/sites/democrats.coronavirus.house.gov/files/2020.05.14%20SSCC-0014393-96_Redacted.pdf); *see also* Email from Paul Alexander, Senior Advisor, Department of Health and Human Services, to Michael Caputo, Assistant Secretary for Public Affairs, Department of Health and Human Services, et al. (May 14, 2022) (SSCC-0014579 – 81) (online at

https://coronavirus.house.gov/sites/democrats.coronavirus.house.gov/files/2020.05.14%20SSCC-0014579-81_Redacted.pdf); Email from Paul Alexander, Senior Advisor, Department of Health and Human Services, to Bill Hall, Deputy Assistant Secretary for Public Affairs, Department of Health and Human Services, et al. (May 13, 2020) (SSCC-0014555 – 60) (online at https://coronavirus.house.gov/sites/democrats.coronavirus.house.gov/files/2020.05.14%20SSCC-0014555-60_Redacted.pdf).

[220] Email from Paul Alexander, Senior Advisor, Department of Health and Human Services, to Michael Caputo, Assistant Secretary for Public Affairs, Department of Health and Human Services, et al. (May 14, 2022) (SSCC-0014579 – 81) (online at online at https://coronavirus.house.gov/sites/democrats.coronavirus.house.gov/files/2020.05.14%20SSCC-0014579-81_Redacted.pdf); *see also* Email from Paul Alexander, Senior Advisor, Department of Health and Human Services, to Bill Hall, Deputy Assistant Secretary for Public Affairs, Department of Health and Human Services, et al. (May 13, 2020) (SSCC-0014555 – 60) (online at https://coronavirus.house.gov/sites/democrats.coronavirus.house.gov/files/2020.05.14%20SSCC-0014555-60_Redacted.pdf); Email from Paul Alexander, Senior Advisor, Department of Health and Human Services, to Michael Caputo, Assistant Secretary for Public Affairs, Department of Health and Human Services (SSCC-0014393 – 96) (online at https://coronavirus.house.gov/sites/democrats.coronavirus.house.gov/files/2020.05.14%20SSCC-0014393-96_Redacted.pdf).

[221] Email from Paul Alexander, Senior Advisor, Department of Health and Human Services, to Michael Caputo, Assistant Secretary for Public Affairs, Department of Health and Human Services (SSCC-0014393 – 96) (online at https://coronavirus.house.gov/sites/democrats.coronavirus.house.gov/files/2020.05.14%20SSCC-0014393-96_Redacted.pdf).

[222] Email from Bill Hall, Deputy Assistant Secretary for Public Affairs, Department of Health and Human Services, to Michael Robinson, Strategic Planning, Department of Health and Human Services, et al. (May 14, 2020) (SSCC-0014782 – 83) (online at https://coronavirus.house.gov/sites/democrats.coronavirus.house.gov/files/2020.05.14%20SSCC-0014782-83_Redacted.pdf).

[223] Centers for Disease Control and Prevention, *Emergency Preparedness and Response: HAN00432* (May 14, 2020) (online at https://emergency.cdc.gov/han/2020/han00432.asp).

[224] Email from Paul Alexander, Senior Advisor, Department of Health and Human Services, to Ryan Murphy, Principal Deputy Assistant Secretary for Public Affairs, Department of Health and Human Services (May 14, 2020) (SSCC-0014807– 10) (online at https://coronavirus.house.gov/sites/democrats.coronavirus.house.gov/files/2020.05.14%20SSCC-0014807-10_Redacted.pdf).

[225] Email from Bill Hall, Deputy Assistant Secretary for Public Affairs, Department of Health and Human Services, to Ryan Murphy, Principal Deputy Assistant Secretary for Public Affairs, Department of Health and Human Services, and Paul Alexander, Senior Advisor, Department of Health and Human Services (May 14, 2020) (SSCC-0014807– 10) (online at https://coronavirus.house.gov/sites/democrats.coronavirus.house.gov/files/2020.05.14%20SSCC-0014807-10_Redacted.pdf).

[226] Hydroxychloroquine—a drug primarily used to prevent and treat malaria that President Trump had championed as a "miracle" treatment for the coronavirus—received emergency use authorization by FDA to treat the coronavirus in March 2020, but the authorization was revoked in June after FDA determined the drug was ineffective as a coronavirus treatment and potentially dangerous. *See, e.g.*, *Trump Tells the Story of a 'Miracle' Cure for COVID-19. But Was It?*, National Public Radio (Apr. 7, 2020) (online at www.npr.org/sections/coronavirus-live-updates/2020/04/07/829302545/trump-tells-the-story-of-a-miracle-cure-for-covid-19-but-was-it); Letter from Rear Admiral Denise M. Hinton, Chief Scientist, Food and Drug Administration, to Gary L. Disbrow, Deputy Assistant Secretary, Department of Health and Human Services (June 15, 2020) (online at www.fda.gov/media/138945/download); Majority Staff, Select Subcommittee on the Coronavirus Crisis, *A "Knife Fight" with the FDA: The Trump White House's Relentless Attacks on FDA's Coronavirus Response* (Aug. 2020) (online at https://coronavirus.house.gov/sites/democrats.coronavirus.house.gov/files/2022.08.24%20The%20Trump%20White

%20House%E2%80%99s%20Relentless%20Attacks%20on%20FDA%E2%80%99s%20Coronavirus%20Response.pdf).

227 Dr. Lara Bull-Otterson, et al., *Hydroxychloroquine and Chloroquine Prescribing Patterns by Provider Specialty Following Initial Reports of Potential Benefit for COVID-19 Treatment — United States, January–June 2020*, Morbidity and Mortality Weekly Report (Sept. 4, 2020) (online at www.cdc.gov/mmwr/volumes/69/wr/mm6935a4.htm).

228 Select Subcommittee on the Coronavirus Crisis, Transcribed Interview of Nina Witkofsky (Feb. 2, 2022) (online at https://coronavirus.house.gov/sites/democrats.coronavirus.house.gov/files/2022.02.02.SSCC%20Interview%20of%20Nina%20Witkofsky%20-%20REDACTED.pdf).

229 Email from Madeleine Hubbard, Special Assistant, Department of Health and Human Services, to Paul Alexander, Senior Advisor, Department of Health and Human Services (June 30, 2020) (SSCC-0007093 – 110) (online at https://coronavirus.house.gov/sites/democrats.coronavirus.house.gov/files/2020.06.30%20SSCC-0007093-110_Redacted.pdf).

230 Select Subcommittee on the Coronavirus Crisis, Transcribed Interview of Henry Walke (Feb. 18, 2022) (online at https://coronavirus.house.gov/sites/democrats.coronavirus.house.gov/files/2022.02.18%20SSCC%20Interview%20of%20Henry%20Walke%2C%20M.D.%20-%20REDACTED.pdf).

231 Email from Paul Alexander, Senior Advisor, Department of Health and Human Services, to Stephen Hahn, Commissioner, Food and Drug Administration, et al.(July 19, 2020) (SSCC-0005448 – 76) (online at https://coronavirus.house.gov/sites/democrats.coronavirus.house.gov/files/07.19.2020%20SSCC-0005448_Redacted.pdf); Email from Paul Alexander, Senior Advisor, Department of Health and Human Services, to Michael Caputo, Assistant Secretary for Public Affairs, Department of Health and Human Services, et al. (Aug. 18, 2020) (SSCC-0016420 – 22) (online at https://coronavirus.house.gov/sites/democrats.coronavirus.house.gov/files/08.18.2020%20SSCC-0016420_Redacted.pdf); Email from Paul Alexander, Senior Advisor, Department of Health and Human Services, to Michael Caputo, Assistant Secretary for Public Affairs, Department of Health and Human Services, et al. (Aug. 30, 2020) (SSCC-0014811 – 12) (online at https://coronavirus.house.gov/sites/democrats.coronavirus.house.gov/files/08.30.2020%20SSCC-0014811_Redacted.pdf).

232 The email attached a journal article regarding hydroxychloroquine prescription trends from October 2019 through March 2020, which Dr. Alexander appeared to mistake for the MMWR itself. *See* Email from Paul Alexander, Senior Advisor, Department of Health and Human Services, to Nina Witkofsky, Senior Advisor, Centers for Disease Control and Prevention, and Michael Caputo, Assistant Secretary for Public Affairs, Department of Health and Human Services (June 29, 2020) (SSCC-0007294 – 305) (online at https://coronavirus.house.gov/sites/democrats.coronavirus.house.gov/files/2020.06.29%20SSCC-0007294-305_Redacted.pdf).

233 Email from Paul Alexander, Senior Advisor, Department of Health and Human Services, to Madeleine Hubbard, Special Assistant, Department of Health and Human Services (June 30, 2020) (SSCC-0006952 – 53) (online at https://coronavirus.house.gov/sites/democrats.coronavirus.house.gov/files/2020.06.30%20SSCC-0006952-53_Redacted.pdf); *see also* Select Subcommittee on the Coronavirus Crisis, Transcribed Interview of Nina Witkofsky (Feb. 2, 2022) (online at https://coronavirus.house.gov/sites/democrats.coronavirus.house.gov/files/2022.02.02.SSCC%20Interview%20of%20Nina%20Witkofsky%20-%20REDACTED.pdf).

234 Email from Madeleine Hubbard, Special Assistant, Department of Health and Human Services, to Michael Caputo, Assistant Secretary for Public Affairs, Department of Health and Human Services, Paul Alexander, Senior Advisor, Department of Health and Human Services, and Brad Traverse, Senior Advisor, Department of Health and Human Services (July 2, 2020) (SSCC-0007178 – 81) (online at https://coronavirus.house.gov/sites/democrats.coronavirus.house.gov/files/2020.07.03%20SSCC-0007178-81_Redacted.pdf).

235 Select Subcommittee on the Coronavirus Crisis, *Transcribed Interview of Charlotte Kent* (Dec. 7, 2020) (online at https://coronavirus.house.gov/sites/democrats.coronavirus.house.gov/files/Kent%20Transcript_Redacted.pdf).

236 *Id.*; Dr. Lara Bull-Otterson, et al., *Hydroxychloroquine and Chloroquine Prescribing Patterns by Provider Specialty Following Initial Reports of Potential Benefit for COVID-19 Treatment — United States, January–June 2020*, Morbidity and Mortality Weekly Report (Sept. 4, 2020) (online at www.cdc.gov/mmwr/volumes/69/wr/mm6935a4.htm).

237 Email from Charlotte Kent, Chief of the Scientific Publications Branch, Centers for Disease Control and Prevention, to Anne Schuchat, Principal Deputy Director, Centers for Disease Control and Prevention (July 27, 2020) (SSCCManual_00071) (online at https://coronavirus.house.gov/sites/democrats.coronavirus.house.gov/files/2020.07.27.2%20SSCCManual-000071_Redacted.pdf); Email from Michael Beach, Associate Director, Centers for Disease Control and Prevention, to Charlotte Kent, Chief of the Scientific Publications Branch, Centers for Disease Control and Prevention, and Henry Walke, Coronavirus Response Incident Manager, Centers for Disease Control and Prevention (July 27, 2020) (SSCCManual-000064 – 70) (online at https://coronavirus.house.gov/sites/democrats.coronavirus.house.gov/files/2020.07.27%20SSCCManual-000064-70_Redacted.pdf).

238 Email from Charlotte Kent, Chief of the Scientific Publications Branch, Centers for Disease Control and Prevention, to Paul Alexander, Senior Advisor, Department of Health and Human Services, et al. (July 28, 2020) (SSCC-0002881 – 88) (online at https://coronavirus.house.gov/sites/democrats.coronavirus.house.gov/files/2020.07.28%20SSCC-0002881-88_Redacted.pdf) (emphasis added).

239 Email from Charlotte Kent, Chief of the Scientific Publications Branch, Centers for Disease Control and Prevention, to Anne Schuchat, Principal Deputy Director, Centers for Disease Control and Prevention (July 27, 2020) (SSCCManual_00071) (online at https://coronavirus.house.gov/sites/democrats.coronavirus.house.gov/files/2020.07.27.2%20SSCCManual-000071_Redacted.pdf); Email from Charlotte Kent, Chief of the Scientific Publications Branch, Centers for Disease Control and Prevention, to Soumya Dunworth, Technical Writer-Editor, Centers for Disease Control and Prevention, et al. (July 28, 2020) (SSCCManual000046 – 50) (online at https://coronavirus.house.gov/sites/democrats.coronavirus.house.gov/files/2020.07.28%20SSCCManual-000046-50_Redacted.pdf).

240 Email from Michael Beach, Associate Director, Centers for Disease Control and Prevention, to Charlotte Kent, Chief of the Scientific Publications Branch, Centers for Disease Control and Prevention, and Henry Walke, Coronavirus Response Incident Manager, Centers for Disease Control and Prevention (July 27, 2020) (SSCCManual-000064 – 70) (online at https://coronavirus.house.gov/sites/democrats.coronavirus.house.gov/files/2020.07.27%20SSCCManual-000064-70_Redacted.pdf).

241 Email from Nina Witkofsky, Senior Advisor, Centers for Disease Control and Prevention, to Ryan Murphy, Principal Deputy Assistant Secretary for Public Affairs, Department of Health and Human Services, et al. (July 28, 2020) (SSCC-0003201 – 02) (online at https://coronavirus.house.gov/sites/democrats.coronavirus.house.gov/files/2020.07.28%20SSCC-0003201-02_Redacted.pdf).

242 Email from Michael Caputo, Assistant Secretary for Public Affairs, Department of Health and Human Services, to Paul Alexander, Senior Advisor, Department of Health and Human Services, and Nina Witkofsky, Senior Advisor, Centers for Disease Control and Prevention (July 27, 2020) (SSCC-0030408 – 09) (online at https://coronavirus.house.gov/sites/democrats.coronavirus.house.gov/files/2020.07.27%20SSCC-0030408-09_Redacted.pdf); Email from Paul Alexander, Senior Advisor, Department of Health and Human Services, to Michael Caputo, Assistant Secretary for Public Affairs, Department of Health and Human Services, et al. (July 27, 2020) (SSCC-0002911 – 13) (online at https://coronavirus.house.gov/sites/democrats.coronavirus.house.gov/files/2020.07.27%20SSCC-0002911-13_Redacted.pdf).

²⁴³ Email from Madeleine Hubbard, Special Assistant, Department of Health and Human Services, to Paul Alexander, Senior Advisor, Department of Health and Human Services (July 31, 2020) (SSCC-0018131 – 33) (online at https://coronavirus.house.gov/sites/democrats.coronavirus.house.gov/files/2020.07.31%20SSCC-0018131-33_Redacted.pdf).

²⁴⁴ Email from Michael Robinson, Strategic Planning, Department of Health and Human Services, to Paul Alexander, Senior Advisor, Department of Health and Human Services (Aug. 6, 2020) (SSCC-0016582) (online at https://coronavirus.house.gov/sites/democrats.coronavirus.house.gov/files/2020.08.06%20SSCC-0016582-84_Redacted.pdf).

²⁴⁵ Email from Paul Alexander, Senior Advisor, Department of Health and Human Services, to Madeleine Hubbard, Special Assistant, Department of Health and Human Services (July 31, 2020) (SSCC-0003286 – 93) (online at https://coronavirus.house.gov/sites/democrats.coronavirus.house.gov/files/2020.07.31%20SSCC-0003286-93_Redacted.pdf); Email from Paul Alexander, Senior Advisor, Department of Health and Human Services, to Michael Caputo, Assistant Secretary of Public Affairs, Department of Health and Human Services, et al. (Aug. 2, 2020) (SSCC-0005298 – 301) (online at https://coronavirus.house.gov/sites/democrats.coronavirus.house.gov/files/2020.08.02%20SSCC-0005298-01_Redacted.pdf); Email from Paul Alexander, Senior Advisor, Department of Health and Human Services, to Madeleine Hubbard, Special Assistant, Department of Health and Human Services, et al. (Aug. 5, 2020) (SSCC-0008029 – 33) (online at https://coronavirus.house.gov/sites/democrats.coronavirus.house.gov/files/2020.08.05%20SSCC-0008029-33_Redacted.pdf); Email from Paul Alexander, Senior Advisor, Department of Health and Human Services, to Nina Witkofsky, Senior Advisor, Centers for Disease Control and Prevention (July 31, 2020) (SSCC-0002931 – 33) (online at https://coronavirus.house.gov/sites/democrats.coronavirus.house.gov/files/2020.07.31%20SSCC-0002931-33_Redacted_0.pdf).

²⁴⁶ Select Subcommittee on the Coronavirus Crisis, Transcribed Interview of Bill Hall (Aug. 31, 2021) (online at https://coronavirus.house.gov/sites/democrats.coronavirus.house.gov/files/2021.08.31%20SSCC%20Interview%20of%20Bill%20Hall%20-%20REDACTED.pdf).

²⁴⁷ Email from Charlotte Kent, Chief of the Scientific Publications Branch, Centers for Disease Control and Prevention, to Michael Iademarco, Director of the Center for Surveillance, Epidemiology, and Laboratory Services, Centers for Disease Control and Prevention (July 28, 2020) (SSCCManual-000059 – 61) (online at https://coronavirus.house.gov/sites/democrats.coronavirus.house.gov/files/2020.07.28%20SSCCManual-000059-61_Redacted.pdf).

²⁴⁸ Transcribed Interview of Charlotte Kent (Dec. 7, 2020) (online at https://coronavirus.house.gov/sites/democrats.coronavirus.house.gov/files/Kent%20Transcript_Redacted.pdf).

²⁴⁹ Select Subcommittee on the Coronavirus Crisis, *Hearing on "The Urgent Need for a National Plan to Contain the Coronavirus"* (July 31, 2020) (online at https://coronavirus.house.gov/subcommittee-activity/hearings/hybridhearing-urgent-need-national-plan-contain-coronavirus).

²⁵⁰ Centers for Disease Control and Prevention, *Media Statement: Study Highlights Importance of CDC Mitigation Strategies* (July 31, 2020) (online at https://stacks.cdc.gov/view/cdc/91341) (noting that CDC's media statement concerning the MMWR article was "Embargoed until: Friday, July 31, 2020, 1 p.m. ET").

²⁵¹ Select Subcommittee on the Coronavirus Crisis, Transcribed Interview of Michael Iademarco (Oct. 29, 2021) (online at https://coronavirus.house.gov/sites/democrats.coronavirus.house.gov/files/2021.10.29%20SSCC%20Interview%20of%20Michael%20Iademarco%20-%20REDACTED.pdf).

²⁵² Select Subcommittee on the Coronavirus Crisis, Transcribed Interview of Robert Redfield (Mar. 17, 2022) (online at https://coronavirus.house.gov/sites/democrats.coronavirus.house.gov/files/2022.03.17%20SSCC%20Interview%20of%20Robert%20Redfield%20-%20REDACTED.pdf).

²⁵³ Email from Paul Alexander, Senior Advisor, Department of Health and Human Services, to Michael Caputo, Assistant Secretary for Public Affairs, Department of Health and Human Services (Aug. 8, 2020) (SSCC-0016509 – 12) (online at

https://coronavirus.house.gov/sites/democrats.coronavirus.house.gov/files/2020.08.08%20SSCC-0016509-12_Redacted.pdf).

[254] Email from Paul Alexander, Senior Advisor, Department of Health and Human Services, to Robert Redfield, Director, Centers for Disease Control and Prevention, et al. (Aug. 8, 2020) (SSCC-0011473 – 77) (online at https://coronavirus.house.gov/sites/democrats.coronavirus.house.gov/files/08.09.2020%20SSCC-0011473_Redacted.pdf) (emphasis in original).

[255] Select Subcommittee on the Coronavirus Crisis, Transcribed Interview of Christine Casey (Oct. 28, 2021) (online at https://coronavirus.house.gov/sites/democrats.coronavirus.house.gov/files/2021.10.28%20SSCC%20Interview%20of%20Christine%20Casey%20-%20REDACTED.pdf).

[256] Select Subcommittee on the Coronavirus Crisis, Transcribed Interview of Henry Walke (Feb. 18, 2022) (online at https://coronavirus.house.gov/sites/democrats.coronavirus.house.gov/files/2022.02.18%20SSCC%20Interview%20of%20Henry%20Walke%2C%20M.D.%20-%20REDACTED.pdf).

[257] Select Subcommittee on the Coronavirus Crisis, Transcribed Interview of Michael Iademarco (Oct. 29, 2021) (online at https://coronavirus.house.gov/sites/democrats.coronavirus.house.gov/files/2021.10.29%20SSCC%20Interview%20of%20Michael%20Iademarco%20-%20REDACTED.pdf).

[258] Select Subcommittee on the Coronavirus Crisis, Transcribed Interview of Christine Casey (Oct. 28, 2021) (online at https://coronavirus.house.gov/sites/democrats.coronavirus.house.gov/files/2021.10.28%20SSCC%20Interview%20of%20Christine%20Casey%20-%20REDACTED.pdf); Email from Christine Casey, Editor of the MMWR Serials, Centers for Disease Control and Prevention, to Director Robert Redfield, Centers for Disease Control and Prevention, et al. (Aug. 9, 2020) (SSCC-0022285 – 89) (online at https://coronavirus.house.gov/sites/democrats.coronavirus.house.gov/files/08.09.2020%20SSCC00022285%20-%20289_Redacted.pdf).

[259] Select Subcommittee on the Coronavirus Crisis, Transcribed Interview of Christine Casey (Oct. 28, 2021) (online at https://coronavirus.house.gov/sites/democrats.coronavirus.house.gov/files/2021.10.28%20SSCC%20Interview%20of%20Christine%20Casey%20-%20REDACTED.pdf).

[260] *Id.*

[261] *Id.*

[262] *Id.*

[263] Select Subcommittee on the Coronavirus Crisis, Transcribed Interview of Charlotte Kent (Dec. 7, 2020) (online at https://coronavirus.house.gov/sites/democrats.coronavirus.house.gov/files/Kent%20Transcript_Redacted.pdf).

[264] Select Subcommittee on the Coronavirus Crisis, Transcribed Interview of Michael Iademarco (Oct. 29, 2021) (online at https://coronavirus.house.gov/sites/democrats.coronavirus.house.gov/files/2021.10.29%20SSCC%20Interview%20of%20Michael%20Iademarco%20-%20REDACTED.pdf).

[265] Select Subcommittee on the Coronavirus Crisis, Transcribed Interview of Robert Redfield (Mar. 17, 2022) (online at https://coronavirus.house.gov/sites/democrats.coronavirus.house.gov/files/2022.03.17%20SSCC%20Interview%20of%20Robert%20Redfield%20-%20REDACTED.pdf).

[266] Centers for Disease Control and Prevention, *Emergency Preparedness and Response: HAN00432* (May 14, 2020) (online at https://emergency.cdc.gov/han/2020/han00432.asp).

[267] Dr. Michelle A. Jorden, et al., *Evidence for Limited Early Spread of COVID-19 Within the United States, January–February 2020*, Morbidity and Mortality Weekly Report (May 29, 2020) (online at www.cdc.gov/mmwr/volumes/69/wr/mm6922e1.htm).

[268] Email from Bill Hall, Deputy Assistant Secretary for Public Affairs, Department of Health and Human Services, to Paul Alexander, Senior Advisor, Department of Health and Human Services, et al. (June 5, 2020) (SSCC-0007790 – 92) (online at https://coronavirus.house.gov/sites/democrats.coronavirus.house.gov/files/2020.06.05%20SSCC-0007790-92_Redacted.pdf).

[269] Mark É. Czeisler, et al., *Public Attitudes, Behaviors, and Beliefs Related to COVID-19, Stay-at-Home Orders, Nonessential Business Closures, and Public Health Guidance — United States, New York City, and Los Angeles, May 5–12, 2020*, Morbidity and Mortality Weekly Report (June 12, 2020) (online at www.cdc.gov/mmwr/volumes/69/wr/mm6924e1.htm); Email from Charlotte Kent, Chief of the Scientific Publications Branch, Centers for Disease Control and Prevention, to Paul Alexander, Senior Advisor, Department of Health and Human Services (June 10, 2020) (SSCC-0022047) (online at https://coronavirus.house.gov/sites/democrats.coronavirus.house.gov/files/2020.06.10%20SSCC-0022047-50_Redacted.pdf); Email from Charlotte Kent, Chief of the Scientific Publications Branch, Centers for Disease Control and Prevention, to Paul Alexander, Senior Advisor, Department of Health and Human Services (June 11, 2020) (SSCC-0022051) (online at https://coronavirus.house.gov/sites/democrats.coronavirus.house.gov/files/2020.06.11%20SSCC-0022051-54_Redacted.pdf).

[270] Erin K. Stokes, et al., *Coronavirus Disease 2019 Case Surveillance — United States, January 22–May 30, 2020*, Morbidity and Mortality Weekly Report (June 12, 2020) (online at www.cdc.gov/mmwr/volumes/69/wr/mm6924e2.htm); Email from Charlotte Kent, Chief of the Scientific Publications Branch, Centers for Disease Control and Prevention, to Paul Alexander, Senior Advisor, Department of Health and Human Services, et al. (June 13, 2020) (SSCC-0022055) (online at https://coronavirus.house.gov/sites/democrats.coronavirus.house.gov/files/2020.06.13%20SSCC-0022055-58_Redacted.pdf).

[271] Dr. Sascha Ellington, et al., *Characteristics of Women of Reproductive Age with Laboratory-Confirmed SARS-CoV-2 Infection by Pregnancy Status — United States, January 22–June 7, 2020*, Morbidity and Mortality Weekly Report (June 26, 2020) (online at www.cdc.gov/mmwr/volumes/69/wr/mm6925a1.htm); Email from Paul Alexander, Senior Advisor, Department of Health and Human Services, to Michael Caputo, Assistant Secretary for Public Affairs, Department of Health and Human Services, et al. (June 25, 2020) (SSCC-0006601 – 03) (online at https://coronavirus.house.gov/sites/democrats.coronavirus.house.gov/files/2020.06.25%20SSCC-0006601-08_Redacted.pdf); Email from Paul Alexander, Senior Advisor, Department of Health and Human Services, to Michael Caputo, Assistant Secretary for Public Affairs, Department of Health and Human Services, and Robert Redfield, Director, Centers for Disease Control and Prevention (June 28, 2020) (SSCC-0007247 – 50) (online at https://coronavirus.house.gov/sites/democrats.coronavirus.house.gov/files/2020.06.28%20SSCC-0007247-52_Redacted.pdf).

[272] Dr. Mark W. Tenforde, et al., *Characteristics of Adult Outpatients and Inpatients with COVID-19 — 11 Academic Medical Centers, United States, March–May 2020*, Morbidity and Mortality Weekly Report (June 30, 2020) (online at www.cdc.gov/mmwr/volumes/69/wr/mm6926e3.htm); Email from Charlotte Kent, Chief of the Scientific Publications Branch, Centers for Disease Control and Prevention, to Paul Alexander, Senior Advisor, Department of Health and Human Services, et al. (June 22, 2020) (SSCCManual-000106) (online at https://coronavirus.house.gov/sites/democrats.coronavirus.house.gov/files/2020.06.22%20SSCCManual-000106-09_Redacted.pdf).

[273] Dr. Lara Bull-Otterson, et al., *Hydroxychloroquine and Chloroquine Prescribing Patterns by Provider Specialty Following Initial Reports of Potential Benefit for COVID-19 Treatment — United States, January–June 2020*, Morbidity and Mortality Weekly Report (Sept. 4, 2020) (online at www.cdc.gov/mmwr/volumes/69/wr/mm6935a4.htm); Email from Paul Alexander, Senior Advisor, Department of Health and Human Services, to Nina Witkofsky, Senior Advisor, Centers for Disease Control and Prevention, and Michael Caputo, Assistant Secretary for Public Affairs, Department of Health and Human Services (June 29, 2020) (SSCC-0007294 – 305) (online at https://coronavirus.house.gov/sites/democrats.coronavirus.house.gov/files/2020.06.29%20SSCC-0007294-305_Redacted.pdf).

[274] Dr. Kiva A. Fischer, et al., *Factors Associated with Cloth Face Covering Use Among Adults During the COVID-19 Pandemic — United States, April and May 2020*, Morbidity and Mortality Weekly Report (July 14,

2020) (online at www.cdc.gov/mmwr/volumes/69/wr/mm6928e3.htm); Email from Paul Alexander, Senior Advisor, Department of Health and Human Services, to Charlotte Kent, Chief of the Scientific Publications Branch, Centers for Disease Control and Prevention, et al. (July 14, 2020) (SSCC-0006018 – 21) (online at https://coronavirus.house.gov/sites/democrats.coronavirus.house.gov/files/2020.07.14%20SSCC-0006018-24_Redacted.pdf); Email from Charlotte Kent, Chief of the Scientific Publications Branch, Centers for Disease Control and Prevention, to Paul Alexander, Senior Advisor, Department of Health and Human Services, et al. (June 10, 2020) (SSCC-0022047 – 48) (online at https://coronavirus.house.gov/sites/democrats.coronavirus.house.gov/files/2020.06.10%20SSCC-0022047-50_Redacted.pdf).

[275] Dr. Hilda Razzaghi, et al., *Estimated County-Level Prevalence of Selected Underlying Medical Conditions Associated with Increased Risk for Severe COVID-19 Illness — United States, 2018*, Morbidity and Mortality Weekly Report (July 24, 2020) (online at www.cdc.gov/mmwr/volumes/69/wr/mm6929a1.htm); Email from Charlotte Kent, Chief of the Scientific Publications Branch, Centers for Disease Control and Prevention, to Paul Alexander, Senior Advisor, Department of Health and Human Services, et al. (July 21, 2020) (SSCCManual-000094) (online at https://coronavirus.house.gov/sites/democrats.coronavirus.house.gov/files/2020.07.21%20SSCCManual-000094-97_Redacted.pdf).

[276] Christine M. Szablewski, et al., *SARS-CoV-2 Transmission and Infection Among Attendees of an Overnight Camp — Georgia, June 2020*, Morbidity and Mortality Weekly Report (July 31, 2020) (online at www.cdc.gov/mmwr/volumes/69/wr/mm6931e1.htm); Email from Charlotte Kent, Chief of the Scientific Publications Branch, Centers for Disease Control and Prevention, to Paul Alexander, Senior Advisor, Department of Health and Human Services, et al. (July 28, 2020) (SSCC-0002881 – 88) (online at https://coronavirus.house.gov/sites/democrats.coronavirus.house.gov/files/2020.07.28%20SSCC-0002881-88_Redacted.pdf); Select Subcommittee on the Coronavirus Crisis, Transcribed Interview of Charlotte Kent (Dec. 7, 2020) (online at https://coronavirus.house.gov/sites/democrats.coronavirus.house.gov/files/Kent%20Transcript_Redacted.pdf).

[277] Dr. Heather Paradis, et al., *Notes from the Field: Public Health Efforts to Mitigate COVID-19 Transmission During the April 7, 2020 Election — City of Milwaukee, Wisconsin, March 13–May 5, 2020*, Morbidity and Mortality Weekly Report (July 31, 2020) (online at www.cdc.gov/mmwr/volumes/69/wr/mm6930a4.htm); Email from Paul Alexander, Senior Advisor, Department of Health and Human Services, to Charlotte Kent, Chief of the Scientific Publications Branch, Centers for Disease Control and Prevention, et al. (July 23, 2020) (SSCC-0005360 – 61) (online at https://coronavirus.house.gov/sites/democrats.coronavirus.house.gov/files/2020.07.27%20SSCC-0005359-63_Redacted.pdf).

[278] Marisa Langdon-Embry, et al., *Notes from the Field: Rebound in Routine Childhood Vaccine Administration Following Decline During the COVID-19 Pandemic — New York City, March 1–June 27, 2020*, Morbidity and Mortality Weekly Report (July 31, 2020) (online at www.cdc.gov/mmwr/volumes/69/wr/mm6930a3.htm); Email from Paul Alexander, Senior Advisor, Department of Health and Human Services, to Charlotte Kent, Chief of the Scientific Publications Branch, Centers for Disease Control and Prevention (July 27, 2020) (SSCC-0005359 – 63) (online at https://coronavirus.house.gov/sites/democrats.coronavirus.house.gov/files/2020.07.27%20SSCC-0005359-63_Redacted.pdf).

[279] Dr. Lindsay Kim, et al., *Hospitalization Rates and Characteristics of Children Aged <18 Years Hospitalized with Laboratory-Confirmed COVID-19 — COVID-NET, 14 States, March 1–July 25, 2020*, Morbidity and Mortality Weekly Report (Aug. 14, 2020) (online at www.cdc.gov/mmwr/volumes/69/wr/mm6932e3.htm); Email from Charlotte Kent, Chief of the Scientific Publications Branch, Centers for Disease Control and Prevention, to Paul Alexander, Senior Advisor, Department of Health and Human Services, et al. (Aug. 6, 2020) (SSCCManual-000032 – 38) (online at https://coronavirus.house.gov/sites/democrats.coronavirus.house.gov/files/2020.08.06%20SSCCManual-000032-38_Redacted.pdf).

[280] Dr. Shana Godfred-Cato, et al., *COVID-19–Associated Multisystem Inflammatory Syndrome in Children — United States, March–July 2020*, Morbidity and Mortality Weekly Report (Aug. 14, 2020) (online at www.cdc.gov/mmwr/volumes/69/wr/mm6932e2.htm); Email from Charlotte Kent, Chief of the Scientific

Publications Branch, Centers for Disease Control and Prevention, to Paul Alexander, Senior Advisor, Department of Health and Human Services, et al. (Aug. 6, 2020) (SSCCManual-000032 – 38) (online at https://coronavirus.house.gov/sites/democrats.coronavirus.house.gov/files/2020.08.06%20SSCCManual-000032-38_Redacted.pdf).

[281] Dr. Laura L. Blaisdell, et al., *Preventing and Mitigating SARS-CoV-2 Transmission — Four Overnight Camps, Maine, June–August 2020*, Morbidity and Mortality Weekly Report (Sept. 4, 2020) (online at www.cdc.gov/mmwr/volumes/69/wr/mm6935e1.htm); Email from Michael Iademarco, Director of the Center for Surveillance, Epidemiology, and Laboratory Services, Centers for Disease Control and Prevention, to Charlotte Kent, Chief of the Scientific Publications Branch, Centers for Disease Control and Prevention (Aug. 27, 2020) (SSCCManual_000017 – 22) (online at https://coronavirus.house.gov/sites/democrats.coronavirus.house.gov/files/2020.08.27%20SSCCManual-000017-22_Redacted.pdf).

[282] Dr. Danae Bixler, et al., *SARS-CoV-2–Associated Deaths Among Persons Aged <21 Years — United States, February 12–July 31, 2020*, Morbidity and Mortality Weekly Report (Sept. 18, 2020) (online at www.cdc.gov/mmwr/volumes/69/wr/mm6937e4.htm); Email from Nina Witkofsky, Acting Chief of Staff, Centers for Disease Control and Prevention, to Charlotte Kent, Chief of the Scientific Publications Branch, Centers for Disease Control and Prevention (Sept. 11, 2020) (SSCCManual_000007 – 10) (online at https://coronavirus.house.gov/sites/democrats.coronavirus.house.gov/files/2020.09.11%20SSCCManual-00007-10_Redacted.pdf); Email from Paul Alexander, Senior Advisor, Department of Health and Human Services, to Michael Caputo, Assistant Secretary of Public Affairs, Department of Health and Human Services, and Nina Witkofsky, Acting Chief of Staff, Centers for Disease Control and Prevention (Sept. 11, 2020) (SSCC-0011333 – 35) (online at https://coronavirus.house.gov/sites/democrats.coronavirus.house.gov/files/2020.09.11%20SSCC-0011333-35_Redacted.pdf); Email from Paul Alexander, Senior Advisor, Department of Health and Human Services, to Madeleine Hubbard, Special Assistant, Department of Health and Human Services, and Michael Caputo, Assistant Secretary of Public Affairs, Department of Health and Human Services (Sept. 11, 2020) (SSCC-0016228 – 35) (online at https://coronavirus.house.gov/sites/democrats.coronavirus.house.gov/files/2020.09.11%20SSCC-0016228-35_Redacted.pdf); Email from Paul Alexander, Senior Advisor, Department of Health and Human Services, to Michael Caputo, Assistant Secretary of Public Affairs, Department of Health and Human Services (Sept. 13, 2020) (SSCC-0011360 – 67) (online at https://coronavirus.house.gov/sites/democrats.coronavirus.house.gov/files/2020.09.13%20SSCC-0011360_Redacted.pdf).

[283] Dr. Noah G. Schwartz, et al., *Adolescent with COVID-19 as the Source of an Outbreak at a 3-Week Family Gathering – Four States, June-July 2020*, Morbidity and Mortality Weekly Report (Oct. 9, 2020) (online at www.cdc.gov/mmwr/volumes/69/wr/mm6940e2.htm); Email from Brett Giroir, Assistant Secretary for Health, Department of Health and Human Services, to Charlotte Kent, Chief of the Scientific Publications Branch, Centers for Disease Control and Prevention, et al. (Oct. 3, 2020) (SSCC-0043296) (online at https://coronavirus.house.gov/sites/democrats.coronavirus.house.gov/files/2020.10.03%20SSCC-0043296_Redacted.pdf).

[284] Dr. Kathleen Dooling, et al., *The Advisory Committee on Immunization Practices' Interim Recommendation for Allocating Initial Supplies of COVID-19 Vaccine – United States, 2020*, Morbidity and Mortality Weekly Report (Dec. 11, 2020) (online at https://cdc.gov/mmwr/volumes/69/wr/mm6949e1.htm); Select Subcommittee on the Coronavirus Crisis, Transcribed Interview of Robert Redfield (Mar. 17, 2022) (online at https://coronavirus.house.gov/sites/democrats.coronavirus.house.gov/files/2022.03.17%20SSCC%20Interview%20of%20Robert%20Redfield%20-%20REDACTED.pdf); Select Subcommittee on the Coronavirus Crisis, Transcribed Interview of Nina Witkofsky (Feb. 2, 2022) (online at https://coronavirus.house.gov/sites/democrats.coronavirus.house.gov/files/2022.02.02.SSCC%20Interview%20of%20Nina%20Witkofsky%20-%20REDACTED.pdf); *see also* Email from Nina Witkofsky, Acting Chief of Staff, Centers for Disease Control and Prevention, to Brett Giroir, Assistant Secretary for Health, Department of Health and Human Services (Dec. 2, 2020) (SSCC-0042789) (online at https://coronavirus.house.gov/sites/democrats.coronavirus.house.gov/files/2020.12.02%20SSCC-0042789_Redacted.pdf).

[285] *See, e.g.*, Select Subcommittee on the Coronavirus Crisis, Transcribed Interview of Charlotte Kent (Dec. 7, 2020) (online at https://coronavirus.house.gov/sites/democrats.coronavirus.house.gov/files/Kent%20Transcript_Redacted.pdf); Select Subcommittee on the Coronavirus Crisis, Transcribed Interview of Anne Schuchat (Oct. 1, 2021) (online at https://coronavirus.house.gov/sites/democrats.coronavirus.house.gov/files/2021.10.01%20SSCC%20Interview%20of%20Anne%20Schuchat%20-%20REDACTED.pdf).

[286] Email from Paul Alexander, Senior Advisor, Department of Health and Human Services, to Nina Witkofsky, Acting Chief of Staff, Centers for Disease Control and Prevention (Aug. 30, 2020) (SSCC-0011064) (online at https://coronavirus.house.gov/sites/democrats.coronavirus.house.gov/files/08.30.2020%20SSCC-0011064_Redacted.pdf).

[287] Email from Paul Alexander, Senior Advisor, Department of Health and Human Services, to Michael Caputo, Assistant Secretary for Public Affairs, Department of Health and Human Services (Sept. 9, 2020) (SSCC0003325 – 26) (online at https://coronavirus.house.gov/sites/democrats.coronavirus.house.gov/files/09.09.2020%20SSCC-0003325-36_Redacted.pdf).

[288] Select Subcommittee on the Coronavirus Crisis, Transcribed Interview of Michael Iademarco (Oct. 29, 2021) (online at https://coronavirus.house.gov/sites/democrats.coronavirus.house.gov/files/2021.10.29%20SSCC%20Interview%20of%20Michael%20Iademarco%20-%20REDACTED.pdf).

[289] Select Subcommittee on the Coronavirus Crisis, Transcribed Interview of Anne Schuchat (Oct. 1, 2021) (online at https://coronavirus.house.gov/sites/democrats.coronavirus.house.gov/files/2021.10.01%20SSCC%20Interview%20of%20Anne%20Schuchat%20-%20REDACTED.pdf).

[290] Letter from Counsel for Kyle McGowan and Amanda Campbell to Chairman James E. Clyburn, Select Subcommittee on the Coronavirus Crisis (June 10, 2022) (online at https://coronavirus.house.gov/sites/democrats.coronavirus.house.gov/files/2022.06.10%20Letter%20to%20Chairman%20Clyburn_Redacted.pdf).

[291] During her transcribed interview with the Select Subcommittee, counsel for HHS instructed Dr. Schuchat not to provide any details regarding the substance of what Mr. Meadows said during this call on the grounds of executive privilege. Select Subcommittee on the Coronavirus Crisis, Transcribed Interview of Anne Schuchat (Oct. 1, 2021) (online at https://coronavirus.house.gov/sites/democrats.coronavirus.house.gov/files/2021.10.01%20SSCC%20Interview%20of%20Anne%20Schuchat%20-%20REDACTED.pdf).

[292] Select Subcommittee on the Coronavirus Crisis, Transcribed Interview of Anne Schuchat (Oct. 1, 2021) (online at https://coronavirus.house.gov/sites/democrats.coronavirus.house.gov/files/2021.10.01%20SSCC%20Interview%20of%20Anne%20Schuchat%20-%20REDACTED.pdf).

[293] Select Subcommittee on the Coronavirus Crisis, Transcribed Interview of Robert Redfield (Mar. 17, 2022) (online at https://coronavirus.house.gov/sites/democrats.coronavirus.house.gov/files/2022.03.17%20SSCC%20Interview%20of%20Robert%20Redfield%20-%20REDACTED.pdf).

[294] Letter from Counsel for Kyle McGowan and Amanda Campbell to Chairman James E. Clyburn, Select Subcommittee on the Coronavirus Crisis (June 10, 2022) (online at https://coronavirus.house.gov/sites/democrats.coronavirus.house.gov/files/2022.06.10%20Letter%20to%20Chairman%20Clyburn_Redacted.pdf).

[295] Select Subcommittee on the Coronavirus Crisis, Transcribed Interview of Anne Schuchat (Oct. 1, 2021) (online at https://coronavirus.house.gov/sites/democrats.coronavirus.house.gov/files/2021.10.01%20SSCC%20Interview%20of%20Anne%20Schuchat%20-%20REDACTED.pdf); Select Subcommittee on the Coronavirus Crisis, Transcribed Interview of Charlotte Kent (Dec. 7, 2020) (online at https://coronavirus.house.gov/sites/democrats.coronavirus.house.gov/files/Kent%20Transcript_Redacted.pdf); Letter

from Counsel for Kyle McGowan and Amanda Campbell to Chairman James E. Clyburn, Select Subcommittee on the Coronavirus Crisis (June 10, 2022) (online at https://coronavirus.house.gov/sites/democrats.coronavirus.house.gov/files/2022.06.10%20Letter%20to%20Chairman%20Clyburn_Redacted.pdf); *see also* Email from Robert Redfield, Director, Centers for Disease Control and Prevention, to Deborah Birx, Coronavirus Response Coordinator, The White House, et al. (May 21, 2020) (SSCC-0042790) (online at https://coronavirus.house.gov/sites/democrats.coronavirus.house.gov/files/2020.05.21%20SSCC-0042790-91_Redacted.pdf); Email from Deborah Birx, Coronavirus Response Coordinator, The White House, to Robert Redfield, Director, Centers for Disease Control and Prevention (May 24, 2020) (SSCC-0035941) (online at https://coronavirus.house.gov/sites/democrats.coronavirus.house.gov/files/2020.05.24%20SSCC-0035941_Redacted.pdf); Email from Brian Harrison, Chief of Staff, Department of Health and Human Services, to Robert Redfield, Director, Centers for Disease Control and Prevention, et al. (May 24, 2020) (SSCC-0035942) (online at https://coronavirus.house.gov/sites/democrats.coronavirus.house.gov/files/2020.05.24%20SSCC-0035942_Redacted.pdf).

[296] Select Subcommittee on the Coronavirus Crisis, Transcribed Interview of Anne Schuchat (Oct. 1, 2021) (online at https://coronavirus.house.gov/sites/democrats.coronavirus.house.gov/files/2021.10.01%20SSCC%20Interview%20of%20Anne%20Schuchat%20-%20REDACTED.pdf).

[297] Select Subcommittee on the Coronavirus Crisis, Transcribed Interview of Christine Casey (Oct. 28, 2021) (online at https://coronavirus.house.gov/sites/democrats.coronavirus.house.gov/files/2021.10.28%20SSCC%20Interview%20of%20Christine%20Casey%20-%20REDACTED.pdf).

[298] Select Subcommittee on the Coronavirus Crisis, Transcribed Interview of Henry Walke (Feb. 18, 2022) (online at https://coronavirus.house.gov/sites/democrats.coronavirus.house.gov/files/2022.02.18%20SSCC%20Interview%20of%20Henry%20Walke%2C%20M.D.%20-%20REDACTED.pdf).

[299] Disclosure from Daniel Wozniczka (Aug. 9, 2022).

[300] Select Subcommittee on the Coronavirus Crisis, Transcribed Interview of Robert Redfield (Mar. 17, 2022) (online at https://coronavirus.house.gov/sites/democrats.coronavirus.house.gov/files/2022.03.17%20SSCC%20Interview%20of%20Robert%20Redfield%20-%20REDACTED.pdf).

[301] *Trump Officials Interfered with CDC Reports on Covid-19*, Politico (Sept. 12, 2020) (online at www.politico.com/news/2020/09/11/exclusive-trump-officials-interfered-with-cdc-reports-on-covid-19-412809).

[302] Email from Paul Alexander, Senior Advisor, Department of Health and Human Services, to Katherine McKeogh, Press Secretary, Department of Health and Human Services, et al. (Sept. 9, 2020) (SSCC-0008026 – 28) (online at https://coronavirus.house.gov/sites/democrats.coronavirus.house.gov/files/2020.09.09%20SSCC-0008026-28_Redacted.pdf).

[303] Email from Charlotte Kent, Chief of the Scientific Publications Branch, Centers for Disease Control and Prevention, to Nina Witkofsky, Acting Chief of Staff, Centers for Disease Control and Prevention, et al. (Sept. 12, 2020) (SSCCManual-000004-06) (online at https://coronavirus.house.gov/sites/democrats.coronavirus.house.gov/files/2020.09.12%20SSCCManual-000004-06_Redacted.pdf).

[304] Select Subcommittee on the Coronavirus Crisis, Transcribed Interview of Nina Witkofsky (Feb. 2, 2022) (online at https://coronavirus.house.gov/sites/democrats.coronavirus.house.gov/files/2022.02.02.SSCC%20Interview%20of%20Nina%20Witkofsky%20-%20REDACTED.pdf).

[305] *See, e.g.*, Email from Paul Alexander, Senior Advisor, Department of Health and Human Services, to Michael Caputo, Assistant Secretary for Public Affairs, Department of Health and Human Services, et al. (Sept. 12, 2020) (SSCC-0022236 – 45) (online at https://coronavirus.house.gov/sites/democrats.coronavirus.house.gov/files/2020.09.13%20SSCC-0022236-45_Redacted.pdf); Email from Paul Alexander, Senior Advisor, Department of Health and Human Services, to

Michael Caputo, Assistant Secretary for Public Affairs, Department of Health and Human Services (Sept. 13, 2020) (SSCC-0015128 – 29) (online at https://coronavirus.house.gov/sites/democrats.coronavirus.house.gov/files/2020.09.13%20SSCC-0015128_Redacted.pdf).

[306] Email from Paul Alexander, Senior Advisor, Department of Health and Human Services, to Michael Caputo, Assistant Secretary for Public Affairs, Department of Health and Human Services (Sept. 13, 2020) (SSCC-0015128 – 29) (online at https://coronavirus.house.gov/sites/democrats.coronavirus.house.gov/files/2020.09.13%20SSCC-0015128_Redacted.pdf).

[307] Email from Michael Caputo, Assistant Secretary for Public Affairs, Department of Health and Human Services, to Paul Alexander, Senior Advisor, Department of Health and Human Services (Sept. 13, 2020) (SSCC-0022236 – 45) (online at https://coronavirus.house.gov/sites/democrats.coronavirus.house.gov/files/2020.09.13%20SSCC-0022236-45_Redacted.pdf).

[308] Email from Michael Iademarco, Director of the Center for Surveillance, Epidemiology, and Laboratory Services, Centers for Disease Control and Prevention, to Charlotte Kent, Chief of the Scientific Publications Branch, Centers for Disease Control and Prevention (Sept. 11, 2020) (SSCCManual-000016) (online at https://coronavirus.house.gov/sites/democrats.coronavirus.house.gov/files/2020.09.11%20SSCCManual-000016_Redacted.pdf); Email from Charlotte Kent, Chief of the Scientific Publications Branch, Centers for Disease Control and Prevention, to Nina Witkofsky, Acting Chief of Staff, Centers for Disease Control and Prevention, and Michael Iademarco, Director of the Center for Surveillance, Epidemiology, and Laboratory Services, Centers for Disease Control and Prevention (Sept. 12, 2020) (SSCCManual-000004 – 06) (online at https://coronavirus.house.gov/sites/democrats.coronavirus.house.gov/files/2020.09.12%20SSCCManual-000004-06_Redacted.pdf); *HHS Spokesman Caputo to Take Medical Leave After Reportedly Accusing CDC Officials of Plotting Against Trump*, CNBC (Sept. 16, 2020) (online at www.cnbc.com/2020/09/16/hhs-spokesman-caputo-to-take-medical-leave-after-reportedly-accusing-cdc-officials-of-plotting-against-trump.html).

[309] Select Subcommittee on the Coronavirus Crisis, Transcribed Interview of Charlotte Kent (Dec. 7, 2020) (online at https://coronavirus.house.gov/sites/democrats.coronavirus.house.gov/files/Kent%20Transcript_Redacted.pdf); Email from Charlotte Kent, Chief of the Scientific Publications Branch, Centers for Disease Control and Prevention, to Nina Witkofsky, Acting Chief of Staff, Centers for Disease Control and Prevention, and Michael Iademarco, Director of the Center for Surveillance, Epidemiology, and Laboratory Services, Centers for Disease Control and Prevention (Sept. 17, 2020) (SSCCManual-000001 – 02) (online at https://coronavirus.house.gov/sites/democrats.coronavirus.house.gov/files/2020.09.17%20SSCCManual-000001-02_Redacted.pdf).

[310] Select Subcommittee on the Coronavirus Crisis, Transcribed Interview of Mark Weber (Aug. 27, 2021) (online at https://coronavirus.house.gov/sites/democrats.coronavirus.house.gov/files/2021.08.27%20SSCC%20Interview%20of%20Mark%20Weber%20-%20REDACTED.pdf).

[311] Food and Drug Administration, *Solicitation for COVID-19 Immediate Surge Public Service Advertising and Awareness Campaign* (Aug. 3, 2020) (online at https://coronavirus.house.gov/sites/democrats.coronavirus.house.gov/files/FDA%20RFP%20%28Immediate%20Surge%29_Redacted.pdf); National Institutes of Health, *Performance Work Statement: COVID 19 Public Health and Reopening America: Public Service Announcements and Advertising Campaign* (online at https://coronavirus.house.gov/sites/democrats.coronavirus.house.gov/files/NIH%20PWS%20%28Short%20Term%29%20-%20NR.pdf); *see also* Government Accountability Office, *COVID-19: Information on HHS's Public Education Campaign* (Mar. 2022) (GAO-22-104724) (online at www.gao.gov/assets/gao-22-104724.pdf).

[312] Letter from Sarah C. Arbes, Assistant Secretary for Legislation, Department of Health and Human Services, to Chairman Raja Krishnamoorthi, Subcommittee on Economic and Consumer Policy (Nov. 13, 2020) (online at https://coronavirus.house.gov/sites/democrats.coronavirus.house.gov/files/2020.11.13%20HHS%20Letter%20to%2

0Krishnamoorthi_Redacted.pdf); Government Accountability Office, *COVID-19: Information on HHS's Public Education Campaign* (Mar. 2022) (GAO-22-104724) (online at www.gao.gov/assets/gao-22-104724.pdf).

[313] Government Accountability Office, *COVID-19: Information on HHS's Public Education Campaign* (Mar. 2022) (GAO-22-104724) (online at www.gao.gov/assets/gao-22-104724.pdf).

[314] *'It's Like Every Red Flag': Trump-Ordered HHS Ad Blitz Raises Alarms*, Politico (Sept. 25, 2020) (online at www.politico.com/news/2020/09/25/trump-hhs-ads-coronavirus-421957).

[315] *White House Snubs Azar, Installs Trump Loyalist Michael Caputo as HHS Spokesperson*, Politico (Apr. 15, 2020) (online at www.politico.com/news/2020/04/15/michael-caputo-azar-hhs-189046) (showing Caputo hired in mid-April 2020); National Institutes of Health, *Performance Work Statement: COVID 19 Public Health and Reopening America: Public Service Announcements and Advertising Campaign* (online at https://coronavirus.house.gov/sites/democrats.coronavirus.house.gov/files/NIH%20PWS%20%28Short%20Term%29%20-%20NR.pdf).

[316] Select Subcommittee on the Coronavirus Crisis, Transcribed Interview of Mark Weber (Aug. 27, 2021) (online at https://coronavirus.house.gov/sites/democrats.coronavirus.house.gov/files/2021.08.27%20SSCC%20Interview%20of%20Mark%20Weber%20-%20REDACTED.pdf).

[317] *Id.*

[318] *Id.*

[319] *Id.*

[320] According to a GAO report, a portion of the funds sent to ASPA under the interagency agreement came from appropriations for CDC under the Paycheck Protection Program and Health Care Enhancements Act. GAO's review "raised questions about whether the expenditures for the public education campaign were consistent with the purposes of the appropriation in the Paycheck Protection Program and Health Care Enhancement Act." GAO noted that CDC later adjusted its accounts to use a different source of funding for the interagency agreement with ASPA. Government Accountability Office, *COVID-19: Information on HHS's Public Education Campaign* (Mar. 2022) (GAO-22-104724) (online at https://gao.gov/assets/gao-22-104724.pdf).

[321] Select Subcommittee on the Coronavirus Crisis, Transcribed Interview of Robert Redfield (Mar. 17, 2022) (online at https://coronavirus.house.gov/sites/democrats.coronavirus.house.gov/files/2022.03.17%20SSCC%20Interview%20of%20Robert%20Redfield%20-%20REDACTED.pdf).

[322] Select Subcommittee on the Coronavirus Crisis, Transcribed Interview of Mark Weber (Aug. 27, 2021) (online at https://coronavirus.house.gov/sites/democrats.coronavirus.house.gov/files/2021.08.27%20SSCC%20Interview%20of%20Mark%20Weber%20-%20REDACTED.pdf); Select Subcommittee on the Coronavirus Crisis, Transcribed Interview of Robert Redfield (Mar. 17, 2022) (online at https://coronavirus.house.gov/sites/democrats.coronavirus.house.gov/files/2022.03.17%20SSCC%20Interview%20of%20Robert%20Redfield%20-%20REDACTED.pdf).

[323] *'It Just Created a Public Relations Nightmare': Inside Michael Caputo's Time at HHS*, Politico (Sept. 16, 2020) (online at https://politico.com/news/2020/09/16/how-michael-caputo-shook-up-hhs-416632).

[324] Select Subcommittee on the Coronavirus Crisis, Transcribed Interview of Mark Weber (Aug. 27, 2021) (online at https://coronavirus.house.gov/sites/democrats.coronavirus.house.gov/files/2021.08.27%20SSCC%20Interview%20of%20Mark%20Weber%20-%20REDACTED.pdf).

[325] *Id.*; Food and Drug Administration, *Solicitation for COVID-19 Immediate Surge Public Service Advertising and Awareness Campaign* (Aug. 3, 2020) (online at https://coronavirus.house.gov/sites/democrats.coronavirus.house.gov/files/FDA%20RFP%20%28Immediate%20Surge%29_Redacted.pdf).

[326] Email from Noah Wills, Contract Specialist, Food and Drug Administration, to Vanessa M. Downes, Senior Director of Contracts, Atlas Research, et al. (Aug. 5, 2020) (online at

https://coronavirus.house.gov/sites/democrats.coronavirus.house.gov/files/2020.08.04%20FDA%20to%20Atlas_Re dacted.pdf); Food and Drug Administration, *Solicitation for COVID-19 Immediate Surge Public Service Advertising and Awareness Campaign* (Aug. 3, 2020) (online at https://coronavirus.house.gov/sites/democrats.coronavirus.house.gov/files/FDA%20RFP%20%28Immediate%20Sur ge%29_Redacted.pdf.

[327] *See* Government Accountability Office, *COVID-19: Information on HHS's Public Education Campaign* (Mar. 2022) (GAO-22-104724) (online at www.gao.gov/assets/gao-22-104724.pdf) (noting the awards were made in September 2020).

[328] Email from Michael Caputo, Assistant Secretary for Public Affairs, Department of Health and Human Services, to Mark Weber, Deputy Assistant Secretary for Public Affairs, Department of Health and Human Services, et al. (July 19, 2020) (SSCC-0005984-85) (online at https://coronavirus.house.gov/sites/democrats.coronavirus.house.gov/files/2020.07.19%20SSCC-0005982-85_Redacted.pdf).

[329] *See* Text Messages between Representative of Atlas Research and Den Tolmor, DD&T (Aug. 31, 2020) (online at https://coronavirus.house.gov/sites/democrats.coronavirus.house.gov/files/2020.08.31%20Tolmor%20and%20Atlas_Redacted.pdf).

[330] *Its's Like Every Red Flag': Trump-Ordered HHS Ad Blitz Raises Alarms*, Politico (Sept. 25, 2020) (online at www.politico.com/news/2020/09/25/trump-hhs-ads-coronavirus-421957).

[331] *Bond.pm to Launch Crowdinvesting Campaign June 25th*, Business Wire (June 7, 2018) (online at www.businesswire.com/news/home/20180607006236/en/Bond.pm-to-Launch-Crowdinvesting-Campaign-June-25th); *Former Trump Campaign Aide: My Russia Ties Are Not Nefarious!*, WIRED (May 25, 2018) (online at www.wired.com/story/former-trump-campaign-aide-my-russia-ties-are-not-nefarious/).

[332] Email from Michael Caputo, Assistant Secretary for Public Affairs, Department of Health and Human Services, to Mark Weber, Deputy Assistant Secretary for Public Affairs, Department of Health and Human Services, et al. (July 19, 2020) (SSCC-0005984-85) (online at https://coronavirus.house.gov/sites/democrats.coronavirus.house.gov/files/2020.07.19%20SSCC-0005982-85_Redacted.pdf).

[333] Email from Representative of Grapeseed Media to Paul Alexander, Senior Advisor, Department of Health and Human Services, et al. (July 20, 2020) (SSCC-0005982-83) (online at https://coronavirus.house.gov/sites/democrats.coronavirus.house.gov/files/2020.07.19%20SSCC-0005982-85_Redacted.pdf); USASpending.gov, *Contract to Atlas Research LLC* (online at www.usaspending.gov/award/CONT_AWD_75F40120C00162_7524_-NONE-_-NONE-) (accessed Oct. 14, 2022).

[334] Select Subcommittee on the Coronavirus Crisis, Transcribed Interview of Mark Weber (Aug. 27, 2021) (online at https://coronavirus.house.gov/sites/democrats.coronavirus.house.gov/files/2021.08.27%20SSCC%20Interview%20of%20Mark%20Weber%20-%20REDACTED.pdf).

[335] *Id.*

[336] *Id.*

[337] *Id.*

[338] *Id.*

[339] *Id.*

[340] Email from Noah Wills, Contract Specialist, Food and Drug Administration, to Young Bang, Chief Growth Officer, Atlas Research, et al. (Aug. 4, 2020) (online at https://coronavirus.house.gov/sites/democrats.coronavirus.house.gov/files/2020.08.04%20FDA%20to%20Atlas_Re dacted.pdf); Co/efficient, *About* (online at https://coefficient.org/about/) (accessed Oct. 14, 2022).

[341] Government Accountability Office, *COVID-19: Information on HHS's Public Education Campaign* (Mar. 2022) (GAO-22-104724) (online at www.gao.gov/assets/gao-22-104724.pdf).

[342] Select Subcommittee on the Coronavirus Crisis, Transcribed Interview of Mark Weber (Aug. 27, 2021) (online at https://coronavirus.house.gov/sites/democrats.coronavirus.house.gov/files/2021.08.27%20SSCC%20Interview%20of%20Mark%20Weber%20-%20REDACTED.pdf); USASpending.gov, *Contract to Atlas Research* (online at www.usaspending.gov/award/CONT_AWD_75F40120C00162_7524_-NONE-_-NONE-).

[343] After the Trump Administration awarded a $250 million contract for a public relations campaign to "defeat despair and inspire hope" amid the pandemic less than two months before the November 2020 presidential election, the Select Subcommittee opened a joint investigation into the objectives for the campaign with the House Committee on Oversight and Reform and the Subcommittee on Economic and Consumer Policy. Letter from Chairwoman Carolyn B. Maloney, Committee on Oversight and Reform, Chairman James E. Clyburn, Select Subcommittee on the Coronavirus Crisis, and Chairman Raja Krishnamoorthi, Subcommittee on Economic and Consumer Policy, to Secretary Alex Azar II, Department of Health and Human Services (Sept. 10, 2020) (online at https://oversight.house.gov/sites/democrats.oversight.house.gov/files/2020-09-10.CBM%20JEC%20RK%20to%20Azar-HHS%20re%20Defeat%20Despair%20Contract.pdf).

[344] Email from Vanessa Downes, Senior Director of Contracts, Atlas Research, to April Brubach, Campaign Director and Contracting Officer's Representative, Department of Health and Human Services, et al. (Sept. 4, 2020) (online at https://coronavirus.house.gov/sites/democrats.coronavirus.house.gov/files/2020.09.04%20Atlas%20to%20HHS_Redacted.pdf).

[345] Subcontractor Agreement between Atlas Research LLC and DD&T Group LLC (Aug. 27, 2020) (online at https://coronavirus.house.gov/sites/democrats.coronavirus.house.gov/files/DDT%20Subcontract_Redacted.pdf).

[346] Email from Mark Chichester, President, Atlas Research, to Vanessa Downes, Senior Director of Contracts, Atlas Research, et al. (Aug. 14, 2020) (online at https://coronavirus.house.gov/sites/democrats.coronavirus.house.gov/files/2020.08.14%20Atlas%20Email_Redacted.pdf). Mr. Weber told the Select Subcommittee that Mr. Tolmor had no prior experience directing or otherwise working on public health campaigns. Select Subcommittee on the Coronavirus Crisis, Transcribed Interview of Mark Weber (Aug. 27, 2021) (online at https://coronavirus.house.gov/sites/democrats.coronavirus.house.gov/files/2021.08.27%20SSCC%20Interview%20of%20Mark%20Weber%20-%20REDACTED.pdf).

[347] Select Subcommittee on the Coronavirus Crisis, Transcribed Interview of Mark Weber (Aug. 27, 2021) (online at https://coronavirus.house.gov/sites/democrats.coronavirus.house.gov/files/2021.08.27%20SSCC%20Interview%20of%20Mark%20Weber%20-%20REDACTED.pdf).

[348] Government Accountability Office, *COVID-19: Information on HHS's Public Education Campaign* (Mar. 2022) (GAO-22-104724) (online at www.gao.gov/assets/gao-22-104724.pdf).

[349] *Id.*

[350] Select Subcommittee on the Coronavirus Crisis, Transcribed Interview of Mark Weber (Aug. 27, 2021) (online at https://coronavirus.house.gov/sites/democrats.coronavirus.house.gov/files/2021.08.27%20SSCC%20Interview%20of%20Mark%20Weber%20-%20REDACTED.pdf).

[351] *Id.*

[352] Email from Michael Caputo, Assistant Secretary for Public Affairs, Department of Health and Human Services, to Madeleine Hubbard, Special Assistant, Department of Health and Human Services, et al. (Sept. 13, 2020) (online at https://coronavirus.house.gov/sites/democrats.coronavirus.house.gov/files/2020.09.14%20HHS%20to%20Atlas_Redacted.pdf).

[353] Email from Tatiana Chelysheva, DD&T, to Ned Riley, Atlas Research, et al. (Sept. 2, 2020) (online at https://coronavirus.house.gov/sites/democrats.coronavirus.house.gov/files/2020.09.03%20DD%26T%20to%20Atlas_Redacted.pdf); Text Messages from Den Tolmor, DD&T, to Representative of Atlas Research (Sept. 7, 2020) (online at

https://coronavirus.house.gov/sites/democrats.coronavirus.house.gov/files/2020.09.07%20Tolmor%20and%20Atlas
_Redacted.pdf); *see also* Text Messages from Den Tolmor, DD&T, to Representative of Atlas Research (Sept. 6, 2020) (online at
https://coronavirus.house.gov/sites/democrats.coronavirus.house.gov/files/2020.09.06%20Tolmor%20and%20Atlas
_Redacted.pdf) (Mr. Tolmor noting he was following Mr. Caputo's recommendation and would "talk to him tomorrow").

[354] Text Messages from Den Tolmor, DD&T, to Representative of Atlas Research (Sept. 6, 2020) (online at https://coronavirus.house.gov/sites/democrats.coronavirus.house.gov/files/2020.09.06%20Tolmor%20and%20Atlas
_Redacted.pdf).

[355] Email from Stefanie Lehmann, Vice President, Atlas Research, to April Brubach, Campaign Director and Contracting Officer's Representative, Department of Health and Human Services, et al. (Sept. 12, 2020) (online at
https://coronavirus.house.gov/sites/democrats.coronavirus.house.gov/files/2020.09.12%20Atlas%20to%20HHS_Re
dacted.pdf).

[356] Email from Madeleine Hubbard, Special Assistant, Department of Health and Human Services, to Stephanie Lehmann, Vice President, Atlas Research, et al. (Sept. 13, 2020) (online at https://coronavirus.house.gov/sites/democrats.coronavirus.house.gov/files/2020.09.14%20HHS%20to%20Atlas_Re
dacted.pdf); Email from Madeleine Hubbard, Special Assistant, Department of Health and Human Services, to Den Tolmor, DD&T, et al. (Sept. 14, 2020) (online at https://coronavirus.house.gov/sites/democrats.coronavirus.house.gov/files/2020.09.14%20Hubbard%20to%20Tolmo
r.pdf).

[357] Select Subcommittee on the Coronavirus Crisis, Transcribed Interview of Mark Weber (Aug. 27, 2021) (online at https://coronavirus.house.gov/sites/democrats.coronavirus.house.gov/files/2021.08.27%20SSCC%20Interview%20o
f%20Mark%20Weber%20-%20REDACTED.pdf).

[358] Email from April Brubach, Campaign Director and Contracting Officer's Representative, Department of Health and Human Services, to Stephanie Lehmann, Vice President, Atlas Research, et al. (Sept. 14, 2020) (online at https://coronavirus.house.gov/sites/democrats.coronavirus.house.gov/files/2020.09.14%20HHS%20to%20Atlas_Re
dacted.pdf).

[359] Select Subcommittee on the Coronavirus Crisis, Transcribed Interview of Mark Weber (Aug. 27, 2021) (online at https://coronavirus.house.gov/sites/democrats.coronavirus.house.gov/files/2021.08.27%20SSCC%20Interview%20o
f%20Mark%20Weber%20-%20REDACTED.pdf).

[360] Public Service Announcement Celebrity Tracker (online at https://coronavirus.house.gov/sites/democrats.coronavirus.house.gov/files/PSA%20Celebrity%20Tracker%20-
%20NR.pdf); Select Subcommittee on the Coronavirus Crisis, Transcribed Interview of Mark Weber (Aug. 27, 2021) (online at https://coronavirus.house.gov/sites/democrats.coronavirus.house.gov/files/2021.08.27%20SSCC%20Interview%20o
f%20Mark%20Weber%20-%20REDACTED.pdf).

[361] Select Subcommittee on the Coronavirus Crisis, Transcribed Interview of Mark Weber (Aug. 27, 2021) (online at https://coronavirus.house.gov/sites/democrats.coronavirus.house.gov/files/2021.08.27%20SSCC%20Interview%20o
f%20Mark%20Weber%20-%20REDACTED.pdf).

[362] *Id.* According to Mr. Weber, Mr. Caputo told him that he did not care if the celebrities supported the president. Mr. Weber stated that he took Mr. Caputo "at his word," despite the content of the PSA Celebrity Tracker. *Id.*

[363] *Compare* Meeting Notes by Atlas Research, COVID-19 PSA & Awareness Campaign (Sept. 29, 2020) (online at https://coronavirus.house.gov/sites/democrats.coronavirus.house.gov/files/2020.09.29%20Atlas%20Notes%20-
%20NR.pdf), *with* Public Service Announcement Celebrity Tracker (online at

https://coronavirus.house.gov/sites/democrats.coronavirus.house.gov/files/PSA%20Celebrity%20Tracker%20-%20NR.pdf).

[364] Public Service Announcement Celebrity Vetting Tracker (Sept. 22, 2020) (online at https://coronavirus.house.gov/sites/democrats.coronavirus.house.gov/files/2020.09.22%20PSA%20Celebrity%20Vetting%20Tracker-%20NR.pdf); *see also* Email from Stephanie Lehmann, Vice President, Atlas Research, to April Brubach, Campaign Director and Contracting Officer's Representative, Department of Health and Human Services, et al. (Sept. 22, 2020) (online at https://coronavirus.house.gov/sites/democrats.coronavirus.house.gov/files/2020.09.22%20Atlas%20to%20HHS_Redacted.pdf) (circulating the tracker to HHS).

[365] Email from Stephanie Lehmann, Vice President, Atlas Research, to April Brubach, Campaign Director and Contracting Officer's Representative, Department of Health and Human Services, et al. (Sept. 17, 2020) (online at https://coronavirus.house.gov/sites/democrats.coronavirus.house.gov/files/2020.09.17%20Altas_PSA%20Celebrity%20Tracker_Redacted.pdf).

[366] Select Subcommittee on the Coronavirus Crisis, Transcribed Interview of Mark Weber (Aug. 27, 2021) (online at https://coronavirus.house.gov/sites/democrats.coronavirus.house.gov/files/2021.08.27%20SSCC%20Interview%20of%20Mark%20Weber%20-%20REDACTED.pdf); Meeting Notes on BCW Draft Messaging Framework (Sept. 17, 2020) (online at https://coronavirus.house.gov/sites/democrats.coronavirus.house.gov/files/2020.09.17%20BCW%20-%20NR.pdf).

[367] Meeting Notes on BCW Draft Messaging Framework (Sept. 17, 2020) (online at https://coronavirus.house.gov/sites/democrats.coronavirus.house.gov/files/2020.09.17%20BCW%20-%20NR.pdf); *'Keep America Great': After Year in Office, Trump Unveils 2020 Campaign Slogan*, NBC News (Mar. 11, 2018) (online at www.nbcnews.com/politics/white-house/keep-america-great-after-year-office-trump-unveils-2020-campaign-n855506).

[368] Select Subcommittee on the Coronavirus Crisis, Transcribed Interview of Mark Weber (Aug. 27, 2021) (online at https://coronavirus.house.gov/sites/democrats.coronavirus.house.gov/files/2021.08.27%20SSCC%20Interview%20of%20Mark%20Weber%20-%20REDACTED.pdf).

[369] *'Its's Like Every Red Flag': Trump-Ordered HHS Ad Blitz Raises Alarms*, Politico (Sept. 25, 2020) (online at www.politico.com/news/2020/09/25/trump-hhs-ads-coronavirus-421957).

[370] Select Subcommittee on the Coronavirus Crisis, Transcribed Interview of Mark Weber (Aug. 27, 2021) (online at https://coronavirus.house.gov/sites/democrats.coronavirus.house.gov/files/2021.08.27%20SSCC%20Interview%20of%20Mark%20Weber%20-%20REDACTED.pdf); *see, e.g.*, Email from Tatiana Chelysheva, DD&T, to Beth Mahan, Atlas Research, et al. (Sept. 21, 2020) (online at https://coronavirus.house.gov/sites/democrats.coronavirus.house.gov/files/2020.09.21%20DD%26T%20to%20Atlas_Redacted.pdf) (Marc Anthony's representative wanted contract language specifying his appearance "will never be used for president [Trump's] campaign").

[371] Atlas Research, COVID-19 PSA & Awareness Campaign (Oct. 1, 2020) (online at https://coronavirus.house.gov/sites/democrats.coronavirus.house.gov/files/2020.10.01%20Atlas%20Report_Redacted.pdf).

[372] Text Messages from Representative of Atlas Research to Den Tolmor, DD&T (Sept. 3, 2020) (online at https://coronavirus.house.gov/sites/democrats.coronavirus.house.gov/files/2020.09.03%20Tolmor%20and%20Atlas%20-%20NR.pdf).

[373] Select Subcommittee on the Coronavirus Crisis, Transcribed Interview of Mark Weber (Aug. 27, 2021) (online at https://coronavirus.house.gov/sites/democrats.coronavirus.house.gov/files/2021.08.27%20SSCC%20Interview%20of%20Mark%20Weber%20-%20REDACTED.pdf). The PSAs were with CeCe Winans and Dennis Quaid. Mr. Weber said that "raw footage" was compiled for a PSA with Rabbi Shulem, but the filming for that PSA was not completed. *Id.*

374 Select Subcommittee on the Coronavirus Crisis, *Hybrid Hearing with Secretary of Health and Human Services Alex M. Azar II*, 116th Cong. (Oct. 2, 2020) (H. Rept.116-124).

375 Letter from Sarah C. Arbes, Assistant Secretary for Legislation, Department of Health and Human Services, to Chairman Raja Krishnamoorthi, Subcommittee on Economic and Consumer Policy (Nov. 13, 2020) (online at https://coronavirus.house.gov/sites/democrats.coronavirus.house.gov/files/2020.11.13%20HHS%20Letter%20to%20Krishnamoorthi_Redacted.pdf); *see also* Select Subcommittee on the Coronavirus Crisis, Transcribed Interview of Mark Weber (Aug. 27, 2021) (online at https://coronavirus.house.gov/sites/democrats.coronavirus.house.gov/files/2021.08.27%20SSCC%20Interview%20of%20Mark%20Weber%20-%20REDACTED.pdf) (listing some of the experts on the review team).

376 Government Accountability Office, *COVID-19: Information on HHS's Public Education Campaign* (Mar. 2022) (GAO-22-104724) (online at www.gao.gov/assets/gao-22-104724.pdf).

377 *Trump Health Aide Pushes Bizarre Conspiracies and Warns of Armed Revolt*, New York Times (Sept. 14, 2020) (online at https://nytimes.com/2020/09/14/us/politics/caputo-virus.html).

378 Select Subcommittee on the Coronavirus Crisis, Transcribed Interview of Jay Butler (Nov. 30, 2021) (online at https://coronavirus.house.gov/sites/democrats.coronavirus.house.gov/files/2021.11.30%20SSCC%20Interview%20of%20Jay%20Butler%20-%20REDACTED.pdf).

379 *Id.*

380 Select Subcommittee on the Coronavirus Crisis, Transcribed Interview of Martin Cetron (May 2, 2022) (online at https://coronavirus.house.gov/sites/democrats.coronavirus.house.gov/files/2022.05.02%20SSCC%20Interview%20of%20Martin%20Cetron%20-%20REDACTED.pdf).

381 Select Subcommittee on the Coronavirus Crisis, Transcribed Interview of Anne Schuchat (Oct. 1, 2021) (online at https://coronavirus.house.gov/sites/democrats.coronavirus.house.gov/files/2021.10.01%20SSCC%20Interview%20of%20Anne%20Schuchat%20-%20REDACTED.pdf); *see also* Select Subcommittee on the Coronavirus Crisis, Transcribed Interview of Kate Galatas (Sept. 30, 2021) (online at https://coronavirus.house.gov/sites/democrats.coronavirus.house.gov/files/2021.09.31%20SSCC%20Interview%20of%20Kate%20Galatas%20-%20REDACTED.pdf).

382 Select Subcommittee on the Coronavirus Crisis, Transcribed Interview of Martin Cetron (May 2, 2022) (online at https://coronavirus.house.gov/sites/democrats.coronavirus.house.gov/files/2022.05.02%20SSCC%20Interview%20of%20Martin%20Cetron%20-%20REDACTED.pdf); *see also* Select Subcommittee on the Coronavirus Crisis, Transcribed Interview of Deborah Birx (Oct. 13, 2021) (online at https://coronavirus.house.gov/sites/democrats.coronavirus.house.gov/files/2021.10.13%20Birx%20TI%20Transcript%20%2B%20Errata.pdf); Andrew G. Atkeson, *Behavior and the Dynamic of Epidemics*, Brookings Papers on Economic Activity (Mar. 24, 2021) (online at www.brookings.edu/bpea-articles/behavior-and-the-dynamic-of-epidemics/); Benjamin Rader, et al., *Mask-Wearing and Control of SARS-CoV-2 Transmission in the USA: A Cross-Sectional Study*, The Lancet (Jan. 19, 2021) (online at https://doi.org/10.1016/S2589-7500(20)30293-4); Kathyrn R. Fair, et al., *Estimating COVID-19 Cases and Deaths Prevented by Non-Pharmaceutical Interventions, and the Impact of Individual Actions: A Retrospective Model-Based Analysis*, Epidemics (June 2022) (online at https://doi.org/10.1016/j.epidem.2022.100557); Michael J. Ahlers, et al., *Non-Pharmaceutical Interventions and COVID-19 Burden in the United States*, medRxiv (Sept. 28, 2021) (online at https://doi.org/10.1101/2021.09.26.21264142); Catalina Amuedo-Dorantes, et al., *Timing of Social Distancing Policies and COVID-19 Mortality: County-Level Evidence from the U.S.*, Journal of Population Economics (Apr. 8, 2021) (online at https://doi.org/10.1007/s00148-021-00845-2); Xiaoshuang Liu, et al., *Differential Impact of NonPharmaceutical Public Health Interventions on COVID-19 Epidemics in the United States*, BMC Public Health (May 21, 2021) (online at https://doi.org/10.1186/s12889-021-10950-2).

383 Select Subcommittee on the Coronavirus Crisis, Transcribed Interview of Deborah Birx (Oct. 12, 2021) (online at

https://coronavirus.house.gov/sites/democrats.coronavirus.house.gov/files/2021.10.12%20Birx%20TI%20Transcript%20%2B%20Errata.pdf); Majority Staff, Select Subcommittee on the Coronavirus Crisis, *The Atlas Dogma: The Trump Administration's Embrace of a Dangerous and Discredited Herd Immunity via Mass Infection Strategy* (June 2022) (online at https://coronavirus.house.gov/sites/democrats.coronavirus.house.gov/files/2022.06.21%20The%20Trump%20Administration%E2%80%99s%20Embrace%20of%20a%20Dangerous%20and%20Discredited%20Herd%20Immunity%20via%20Mass%20Infection%20Strategy.pdf).

[384] Select Subcommittee on the Coronavirus Crisis, *Press Release: Ahead of Hearing, Select Subcommittee Releases New Evidence of Trump Administration's Prioritization of Politics over Public Health* (June 23, 2022) (online at https://coronavirus.house.gov/news/press-releases/clyburn-trump-birx-atlas-emails-transcript-pandemic-response).

[385] Majority Staff, Select Subcommittee on the Coronavirus Crisis, *A "Knife Fight" with the FDA: The Trump White House's Relentless Attacks on FDA's Coronavirus Response* (Aug. 2022) (online at https://coronavirus.house.gov/sites/democrats.coronavirus.house.gov/files/2022.08.24%20The%20Trump%20White%20House%E2%80%99s%20Relentless%20Attacks%20on%20FDA%E2%80%99s%20Coronavirus%20Response.pdf).

[386] *Americans' Trust in Scientists, Other Groups Declines*, Pew Research Center (Feb. 15, 2022) (online at https://pewresearch.org/science/2022/02/15/americans-trust-in-scientists-other-groups-declines/).

[387] *Only 44 Percent of Americans Trust What the CDC Has Said About COVID: Poll*, Newsweek (Jan. 23, 2022) (online at https://newsweek.com/only-44-percent-americans-trust-what-cdc-has-said-about-covid-poll-1671988); Hart Research Associates/Public Opinion Strategies, *Study #220027: NBC News Survey* (Jan. 2022) (online at https://s3.documentcloud.org/documents/21184709/220027-nbc-news-january-poll.pdf).

[388] Kaiser Family Foundation, *Press Release: COVID-19 Misinformation Is Ubiquitous : 78% of the Public Believes or Is Unsure About At Least One False Statement, and Nearly a Third Believe At Least Four of Eight False Statements Tested* (Nov. 8, 2021) (online at https://kff.org/coronavirus-covid-19/press-release/covid-19-misinformation-is-ubiquitous-78-of-the-public-believes-or-is-unsure-about-at-least-one-false-statement-and-nearly-at-third-believe-at-least-four-of-eight-false-statements-tested/); *see, e.g., Just 12 People Are Behind Most Vaccine Hoaxes on Social Media, Research Shows*, National Public Radio (May 14, 2021) (online at https://npr.org/2021/05/13/996570855/disinformation-dozen-test-facebooks-twitters-ability-to-curb-vaccine-hoaxes).

www.ingramcontent.com/pod-product-compliance
Lightning Source LLC
Chambersburg PA
CBHW081159270326
41930CB00014B/3211